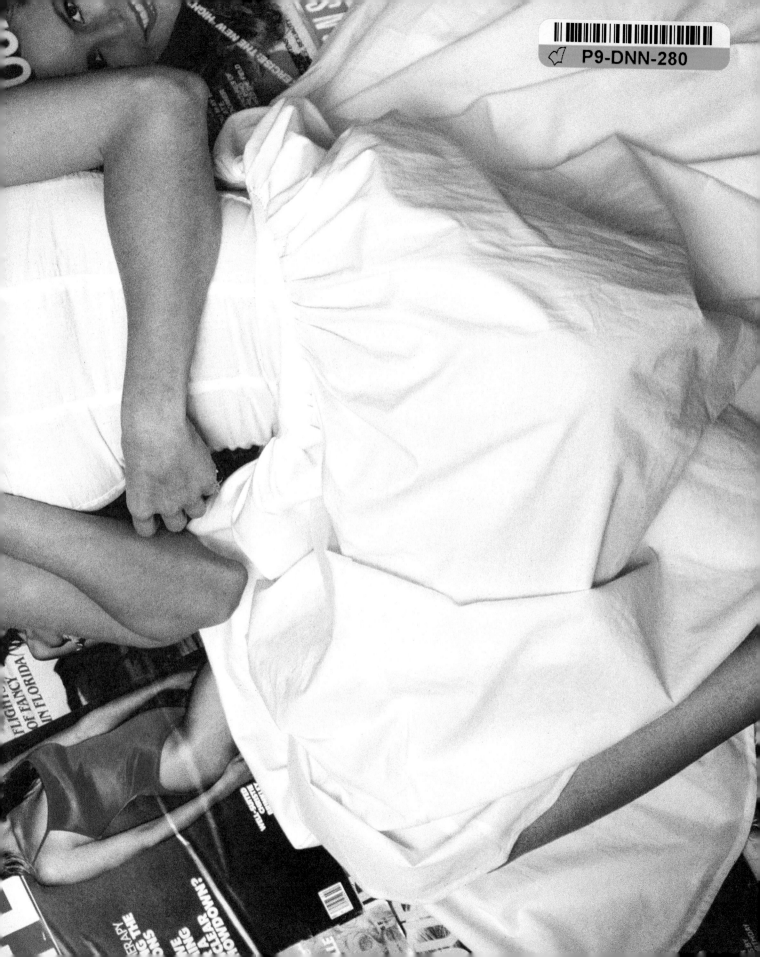

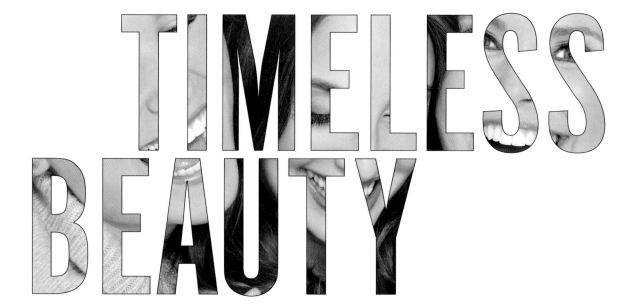

TIMELESS BEAUTY

Sailor, Alexa Ray, me, and don't forget my "Songhine," Jack Paris (not pictured here)

TIMELESS BEAUTY

OVER 100 TIPS, SECRETS, AND SHORTCUTS TO LOOKING GREAT

Christie Brinkley

with Sally Wadyka

GRAND CENTRAL
Life & Style

NEW YORK • BOSTON

DESIGNED BY 8 ½

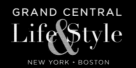

Jacket and case photo by Andrew Macpherson/CPI Syndication
Cover and book design by Eight and a Half, NYC
8point5.com

Front endpaper photo is copyright ©Douglas Kirkland
Back endpaper photo is by Anna Gunselman

Illustrations by Amy van Luijk
Additional copyright information can be found on pages 198 and 199.

Grand Central Life & Style
Hachette Book Group
1290 Avenue of the Americas
New York, NY 10104
www.GrandCentralLifeandStyle.com

Printed in the United States of America

WOR

First Edition: November 2015

10 9 8 7 6 5 4 3 2 1

Grand Central Life & Style is an imprint of Grand Central Publishing.
The Grand Central Life & Style name and logo are trademarks of Hachette Book Group, Inc.

The Hachette Speakers Bureau provides a wide range of authors for speaking events.
To find out more, go to www.HachetteSpeakersBureau.com or call (866) 376-6591.

The publisher is not responsible for websites (or their content)
that are not owned by the publisher.

Library of Congress Cataloging-in-Publication Data has been applied for.

ISBN: 978-1-4555-8794-0 (hardcover) / ISBN: 978-1-4555-6593-1 (hardcover—Barnes & Noble signed edition) / ISBN: 978-1-4555-9390-3 (hardcover—signed edition) / ISBN: 978-1-4789-6053-9 (downloadable audio) / ISBN: 978-1-4555-8792-6 (e-book)

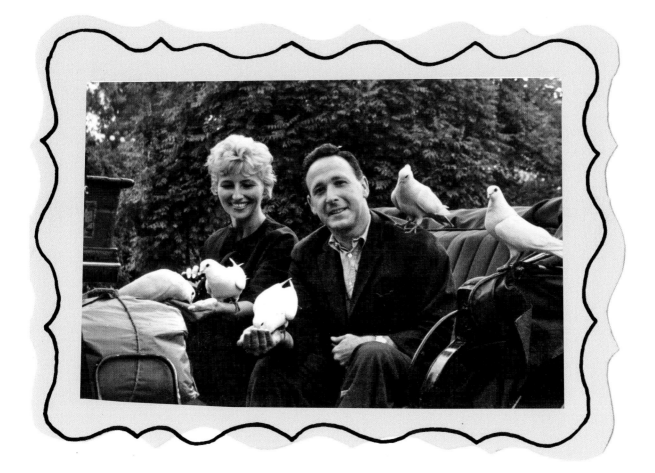

To my wonderful mom,

Marjorie Marie Brinkley,

whose greatest beauty was her ability
to make everyone she met feel
special, appreciated, loved, and beautiful too.

And to my dad,

Donald Alan Brinkley,

who spent every second of his life
doing that for my mom.

Also to everyone who makes it their mission
to spread kindness, compassion,
light, and love in the form of support,
compliments, a helping hand, and a sweet smile.

CONTENTS

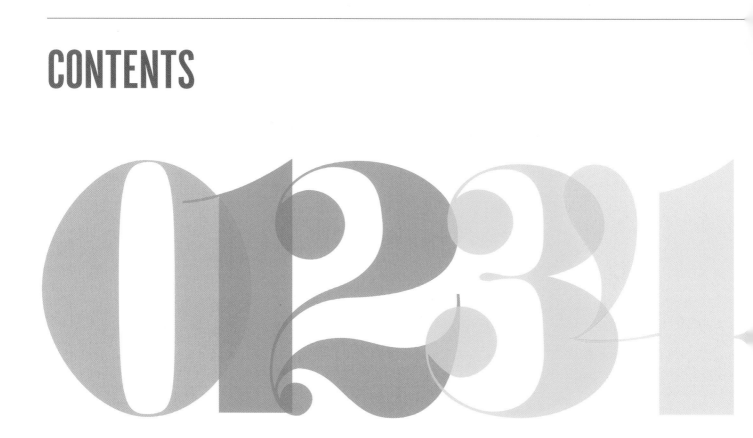

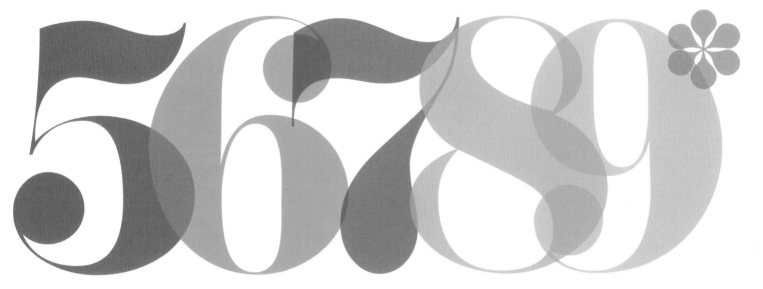

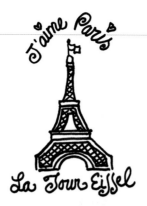

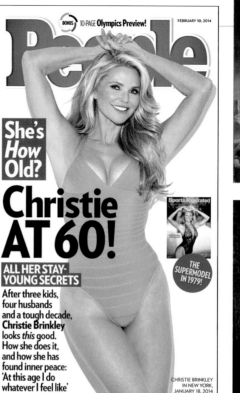

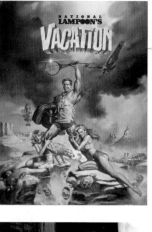

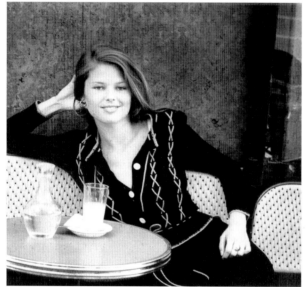

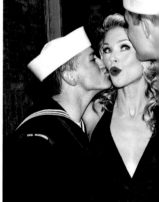

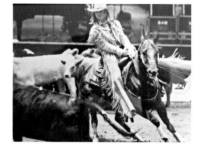

Welcome

OO LA LA! I was asked to become a model while living in Paris, working as an "artiste." This was way back in the day, when the thinking was that at my ripe old age of nineteen, I might already be too old for the business. The rule of thumb was "This business will chew you up and spit you out long before you turn thirty!"

Well, ten years later, at twenty-nine years of age and miraculously still in possession of a bustling modeling career, I wrote my first beauty book. I

wanted to share what I had learned growing up on the beach in Malibu and what I'd picked up from a fascinating industry that had taken me from California surfer girl to cover girl.

I NEVER imagined that I would be writing another beauty book thirty years later, or that I would STILL be modeling! But here I am today, doing BOTH!

The idea to write this book was prompted by the fact that *People* magazine celebrated my Big Six-O by placing me on their cover in a bathing suit.

At the same time, *Sports Illustrated* (who made me the first model to be on the cover of their legendary swimsuit edition three times in a row) was celebrating the fiftieth anniversary of their bestselling franchise, and they coaxed me into a bikini for a TV commercial.

This double whammy of exposure garnered quite a lot of attention! "I'll have what she's having," article after article exclaimed, while proclaiming "60's the New 30!" And those articles got me thinking: What am I doing right that

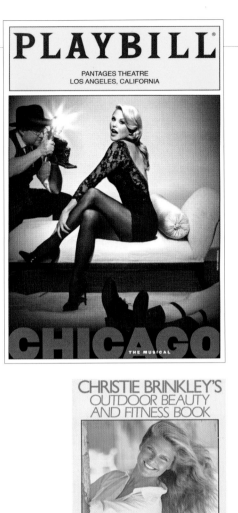

PLAYBILL®

PANTAGES THEATRE
LOS ANGELES, CALIFORNIA

CHICAGO
THE MUSICAL

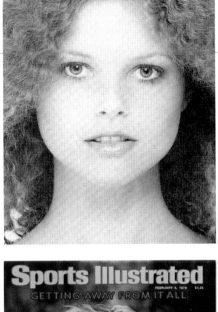

CHRISTIE BRINKLEY'S
OUTDOOR BEAUTY
AND FITNESS BOOK

BY CHRISTIE BRINKLEY

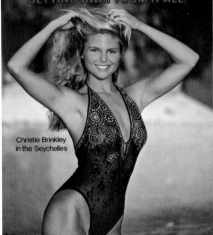

Sports Illustrated
FEBRUARY 5, 1979 $1.25
GETTING AWAY FROM IT ALL

Christie Brinkley
in the Seychelles

Sports Illustrated
FEBRUARY 4, 1980 $1.25
Islands
in the
Sun

Christie Brinkley
Brightens
The British Virgins

Sports Illustrated
FEBRUARY 9, 1981 $1.50
FLIGHTS
OF FANCY
IN FLORIDA

Christie Brinkley
on Captiva

I could share with other people? And if I keep it up, who knows? I could be writing my third beauty book in another thirty years. Maybe ninety will be the new sixty!

I know that I am not unique just because I look "good for my age." Women of all ages are looking and feeling better than the number that's supposed to define them (which many don't reveal so we don't know they look great for sixty and actually believe them when they say they're fifty-five, fifty-two, or forty-nine!).

Thanks to healthy diets, exercise, and youth-enhancing beauty tricks, they can get away with lying about their age. But I say proclaim it and help redefine the way we think about the numbers! Now, having been part of the modeling industry for over forty years, I find myself in a unique position. During that time, I have had the great privilege of working with the best of the best in the worlds of beauty and style. And I simply want to share my good luck and everything I've learned with all of you.

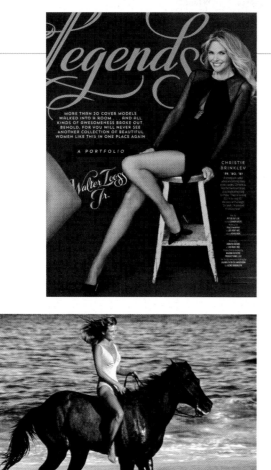

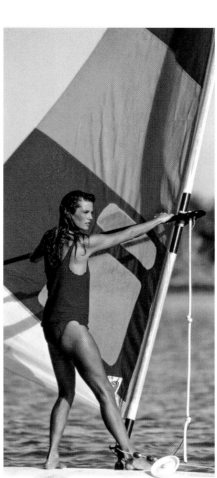

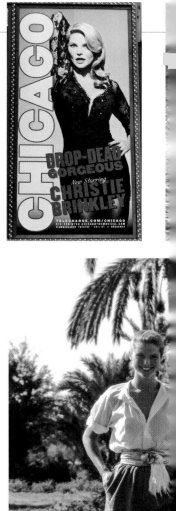

Our world thrives on perfection, and every celebrity has a collection of airbrushed photographs to prove it. But I think it's important to remember that imperfect is sometimes the most perfect. It's an attitude the beauty and modeling worlds are embracing more and more, and I applaud that. I hope this book helps us all learn to love what makes each of us unique and to celebrate it. Because someone can have the most perfect face, body, hair, outfit—but without passion, curiosity, kindness, and compassion, that

sort of beauty is only of fleeting interest.

I am also practical enough to know that when heading out to make the world a better place, you want to look your best. And I hope that's where this book comes in...as a way to help you shine your brightest as you fill the pages of your life with value and meaning and the REALLY important stuff—family, friends, laughter, and LOVE!

I truly believe that everyone is beautiful in her own way. But we can all use a little advice that makes us feel prettier

or maybe a bit more confident. It's like spit on a seashell—beauty loves a little polish! So I hope from this book you will learn the tricks of the trade plus some of my own tried-and-true tips—from recipes to fuel your day, to shortcuts I've learned from the top hairdressers, makeup artists, colorists, wardrobe stylists, and dermatologists that will make you feel like a million bucks!

Basically I hope that after reading this book, you will look in the mirror and smile (that has always been my

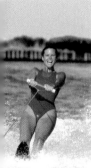

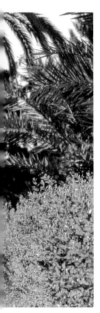

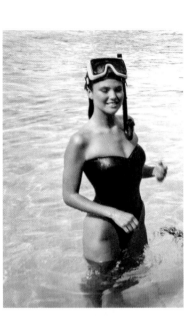

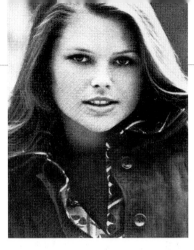

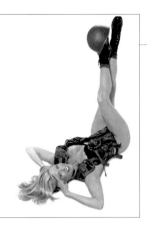

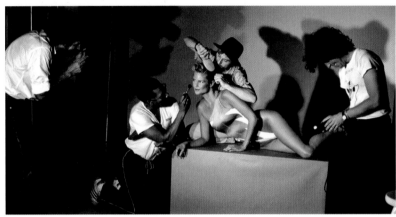

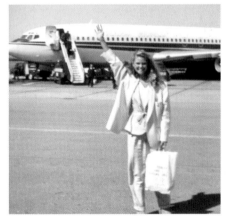

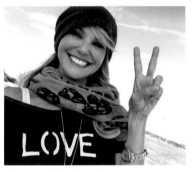

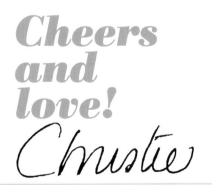

number one beauty secret). A smile has incredible power. It expresses kindness, compassion, generosity, and love without a single word. It can turn a stranger into a friend, it releases powerful feel-good hormones that make you feel happy, and it lights up a room, and your face, in the most delightful way. So smile! We all know that when you feel good, you look good—and that's a legendary formula guaranteed to make you SMILE!

Cheers and love!

Christie

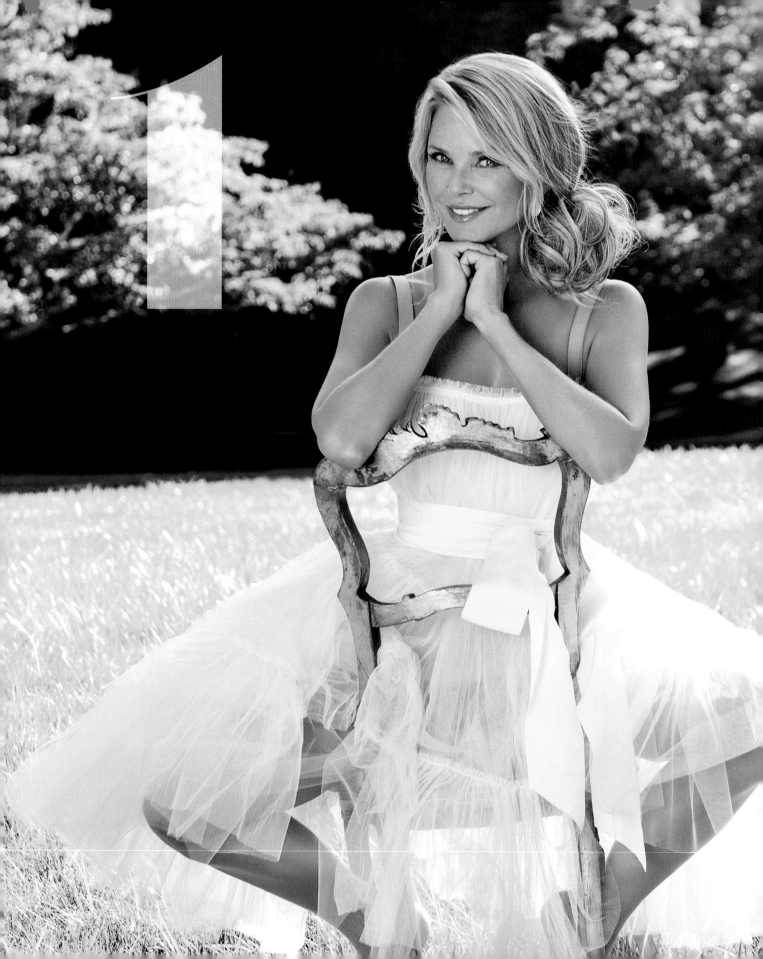

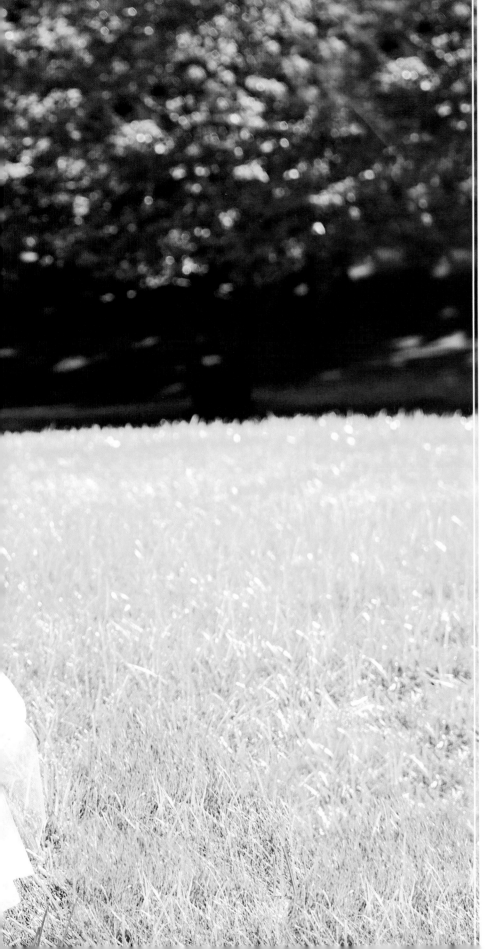

POSITIVELY BEAUTIFUL

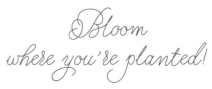

Bloom where you're planted!

Hello Beautiful!

Thank you for picking up my book. A very smart move.

Wow! Smart and beautiful, that's a lethal combination!

Seriously, I want to start this book by reminding you that you are already beautiful, you always have been and always will be. And I truly believe that everything you need to lead a beautiful, healthy, happy and fulfilling life is already inside you. This book is going to keep reminding you of that, and hopefully put you in touch with your inner voice — the one that can be so critical and demanding, and turn that voice into your own best friend, coach and cheerleader!

I want to help you uncover your own amazing positive power, and that will help make your unique beauty shine EVEN brighter. The chapter on nutrition will help you make better choices to fuel your dreams — and health. The chapters on skin and hair, make up and fashion will provide you with tips, tricks and perhaps a little tweak from one of the treatments described by my team of experts to help you look great!

I hope this book will inspire you to get stronger, fitter, and leaner so you are ready to take on any project, challenge, or occasion as a caring and active member of the world around you. I guess you could say that I want you to find ways to leave a beautiful mark, change the world, make it better—and feel beautiful while you're doing it. (By the way, you will never look more beautiful than when you are helping others!)

For as long as I've been part of the modeling industry (forty years and counting!), people have been asking me to reveal my "beauty secrets." I hear questions all the time like, "What makeup do you use? What's your skin care routine? How do you stay so young looking? [Why, thank you!] What do you do for exercise?" And I promise that these pages will answer all those questions and that you will learn LOTS of secrets, tricks, and tips for looking and feeling good. In fact, by the time you're finished reading this book, you'll pretty much know everything I know when it comes to fashion, beauty, food, and fitness! And while I am not a doctor, nutritionist, fitness guru, hairstylist, or makeup artist, I have had access to many of the best in these fields. As you read through these chapters, I'll introduce you to several experts whose opinions I trust, and ask them to share their wisdom with you.

I'll admit that we're going to cover a lot of so-called "superficial" ground on

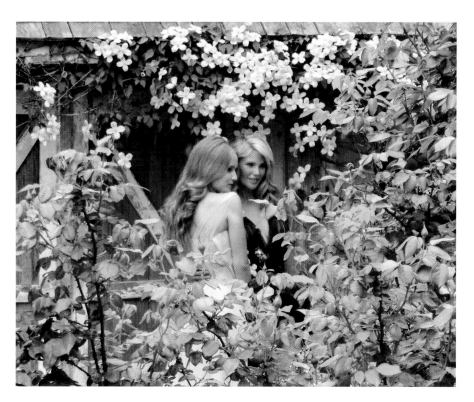

these pages—and hopefully balance it out with some ways to buff up your inner beauty. But c'mon, we all want to put our best face forward, and I promise to show you how to do that while making it seem as effortless as possible. Because seriously, these days, thanks to all the social media sites, every day is like a photo shoot—and you want to be prepared!

But all these skin care and makeup tips are just one part of what I call full-spectrum beauty. And that's the kind of beauty we are ultimately after. That's the kind of beautiful that happens when inner beauty and outer beauty align. Full-spectrum beauty is that special something that makes a person's eyes sparkle with humor, that makes a smile genuine and kind; it's something in a warm, hearty laugh that lights up

a room. It's an open hand and heart, lending support to those in need. Full-spectrum beauty is the part of beautiful that comes from a person's soul. People have searched the world over to find the fountain of youth, but guess what—it's right inside each and every one of us, in our own heart and soul! THAT is the fountain of youth because that's the part of beauty that will never fade. That's the beauty you want to cultivate.

Let your open heart shine, and, along with a little confidence-boosting polish from the tips in this book, I promise you will positively rule, you unique and extraordinary, one-of-a-kind beauty you! Go forth and make this world a more beautiful place. (And hey, we all know it's easier to change the world on good hair days, so read on!)

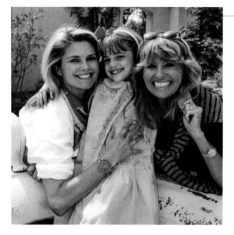

Change your mind

(and the rest will follow)

Now that we all have our hearts in the right place, let's talk about the most powerful muscle in your body—your mind! Well, I'm not sure it's really a muscle per se, but its power to influence our health is truly awesome. The mind-body connection is one of the most potent and woefully underused forces we have at our disposal at all times. But I promise that if you take the time to harness it, you will reap countless rewards. This is something you can work into so many aspects of your life. For example, when I'm exercising, I always reach for the muscle I'm working out and just touch it. My brain tells that muscle, "Hey, we're focused on making you stronger." I've done this instinctively for years, but there's some evidence to back up my instinct. Making that connection between your brain and your muscles will actually help you get a more effective workout. You'll be surprised what a difference it makes!

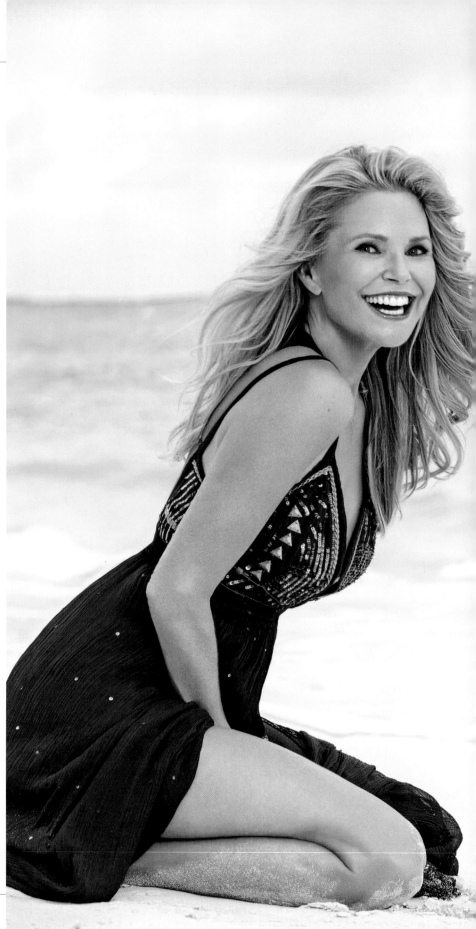

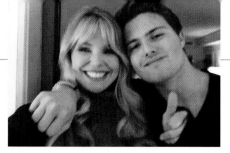

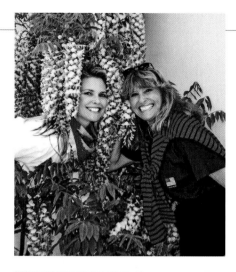

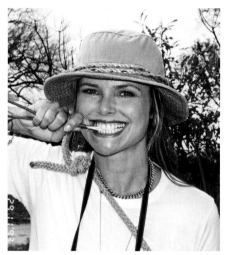

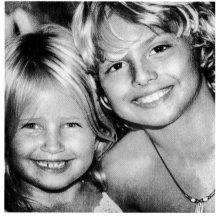

QUICK TIP
BRIGHTEN UP YOUR SMILE

Keep your smile healthy by getting regular checkups, and by brushing and flossing every day. I like **Pepsodent** and **Crest Pro-Health Whitening** toothpastes as a gentle way to keep my pearly whites sparkling. **Oral-B** makes my favorite toothbrushes, and I always mix it up with different-shaped brushes since some are better at getting to those back teeth and some are kinder to the gums. I also love water picks and toothpicks with the miniature bottle brush on one end.

The power of a smile

If you've ever read any interviews with me, you'll know I always say that my best beauty secret is smiling. And not just for the reason you might think. Sure, someone who's smiling will always look prettier, happier, and more approachable than someone who is frowning. But the power of a smile goes deeper than that. Research has shown that smiling doesn't just make you *look* happy, it actually makes you *feel* happy. That's right! No matter what's going on in your life, if you simply put your lips into a smiling position, it can release enough endorphins (the same feel-good chemicals released when we exercise) to improve your mood. Studies have been done measuring the effects of both genuine and forced smiles. And results show that even those who were faking the happy expression had lower heart rates and reported feeling less stressed than those who weren't smiling. (So it's worth faking a smile even when you aren't feeling it, because soon you will!) Plus, smiling is contagious. As they say, smile and the world smiles with you.

Turns out, frowning can affect your attitude too. Frowning sends signals to your brain that actually depress your mood. In an interesting study, researchers found that Botox can help relieve depression because apparently, if you can't frown, your body does not signal the release of the downer hormones. (To be clear: I'm certainly not saying you need to get Botox in order to be happy—I'm also not judging you if you do—but just pay attention to your expressions and try to smile much more often than you frown.)

Words can also influence your health. Your body is always listening to your inner voice, so make sure you are always sending it positive messages. My mom taught me the importance of this early on. When I was just a kid, she would correct me if I ever said the forbidden, "That makes me sick." She was convinced I could actually make myself sick that way! Same thing with "I can't." My mom taught me to say "I choose not to" instead. The point was to reinforce that I had the power to choose and to be in control of those choices. That is how I've always tried to live my life—think positive, feel positive. That's what I've tried to teach my children, and it's exactly the message I hope to convey to you throughout this book.

A positive attitude

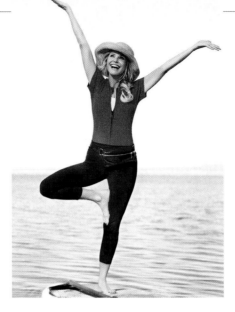

So now that we are all smiling, it's the perfect time to talk about how to cultivate a great attitude to go along with that sexy smile. As far as I'm concerned, there really is nothing more important to health, beauty, and your overall well-being than keeping a positive attitude. It's a given that everyone will face challenges in their lives, so we may as well learn from our struggles, challenges, and mistakes. You know that expression "Smooth seas do not make skillful sailors"? Well, it's true. You learn so much about yourself and others during tough times. And what really defines us is how we get back up after we fall. I have learned to thank the problems I've had for helping me make the acquaintance of a part of me I never knew. "Hello there, strong lady! Nice to meet you! Where'd you come from? Well, your timing is impeccable because I need you right now." (Isn't it nice to know you have that strength when you need it?)

There are certainly times during which it's harder than others to stay positive and find any shred of silver lining. When my parents were ill, it was excruciating for me to see them suffering, and I didn't really know how to cope with that. When I count my blessings, my family always comes first, and two of my most cherished people were in pain. But I also knew that I needed to be there for my kids (my other blessings). So I would focus on doing what I could for my parents and then go home and appreciate that I had my children and that they were healthy. It was also a reminder that life goes so quickly, and that every day that we have each other and have our health is something to celebrate.

I know a lot of women have also gone through struggles similar to those I had with unhappy marital situations and divorce. It can absolutely drain your energy and feel almost impossible to navigate—especially when there are kids involved. You feel very alone, and having to put on a brave face for your children only increases that sense of isolation. I direct a lot of women to a website called One Mom's Battle (onemomsbattle.com). Going on there and reading about what others are going through makes you realize you're not alone, and that no matter what feelings you're having, you're not crazy! You can get a lot of community support that way, and even do it anonymously if you prefer. I also believe that laughter with friends is the number one cure-all. When you are going through trying times, don't be afraid to reach out to your friends. It's so important!

And I think it's good to acknowledge that sometimes we can actually find positive motivation in these very negative situations. And that's not a bad thing! I went through a very public divorce, and when I would read the ugly comments written about me online, it inspired me to really pull myself together and make those naysayers eat their words. For a brief moment, if you need to use something negative to motivate you to do something positive, that's okay. I say, do whatever it takes to not just lie in bed and feel sorry for yourself. As they always say, "What doesn't kill you makes you stronger," and that's true as long as you learn from it, grow, and move on to become more empathetic, compassionate, and stronger than ever.

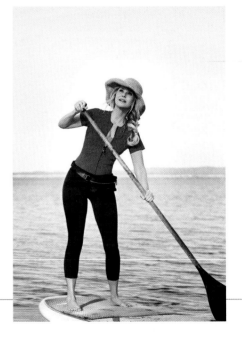

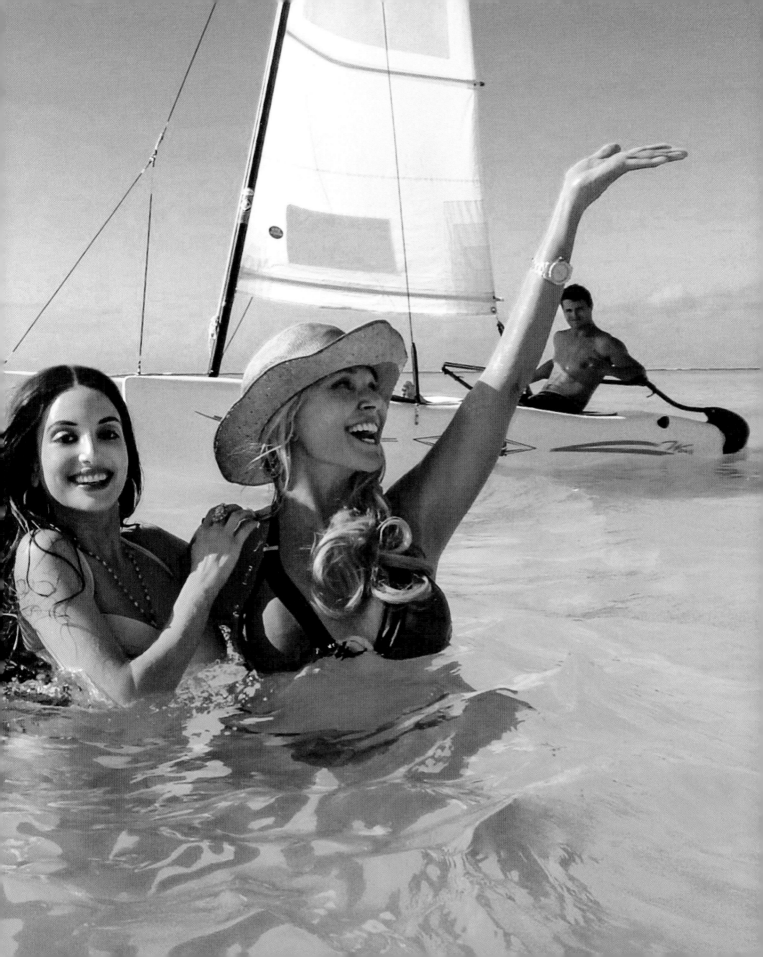

Find some inner peace

Taking good care of yourself—through good times and trying ones—must include time for your spirit too. Meditation is a great example of the power of our mind-body connection. Study after study has found remarkable physical and emotional benefits that can be gained by simply spending a few minutes every day clearing your mind. You can lower your blood pressure, reduce your risk of heart disease and some cancers, sleep better, and even relieve symptoms of conditions like asthma. And you don't have to get all New Agey in order to do it.

Meditation can be as simple as just sitting quietly and focusing on your breathing for a few minutes. Try to clear your mind, and as it wanders and thoughts come in and out, acknowledge them, but then bring your focus back to your breath. You can count your breaths (inhale on one, exhale on two, and so on) or repeat a word or mantra with every exhale (like "peace" or "love") to help you stay more focused. I've been meditating on and off since I was thirteen, but I must admit, I am not a good dedicated meditator. I am more of what I like to call a "meditation opportunist." I pull it out in times of trouble, trials, and tribulations, and on bumpy flights! I add Ujjayi breath and hand *mudras* and it keeps me from grabbing my neighbor's arm with every bump on the plane. I don't even care if I look silly doing it, because it really helps me. It is also invigorating when I'm jet-lagged—twenty minutes of meditating is like getting a couple of hours of sleep.

I also believe that you can get many of these same benefits from meditating on the move. In fact, when people have asked me how I've dealt with some of the challenges I have been lucky enough to learn from, that is what I tell them. I love to grab a camera and walk around looking for beauty. I find beauty everywhere—from the beach to the woods to the cracks in a city sidewalk! It fills me up with gratitude and joy, so that there's just no room for negative thoughts to fit in. I am transported by the magic and light, and I literally feel enlightened, both physically and spiritually, by the beauty. There's a saying: "When you seek beauty in people, and in all things, you will not only find it, you will become it." I do believe that's true. And I do believe that comes from having a feeling of gratitude. So since we're talking beauty secrets here, always remember: a grateful heart is worth a thousand lipsticks!

Throughout all my good times and bad times—whether I've been deliriously happy, totally stressed out, or even downright miserable—I've worked really hard to see the glass as more than half full. Most of the time, it's near to overflowing! Much of my optimism, positivity, and strength comes from being surrounded by my family. My three beautiful children—Alexa Ray, Jack Paris, and Sailor Lee—are my greatest blessings and they bring me my greatest joy. Spending time with them is guaranteed to put a smile on my face!

If you follow me on Instagram, you'll know that I'm constantly posting little quotes and sayings—about 99 percent of which have something to do with an optimistic outlook on life. They're great little daily reminders to look on the bright side and focus on the many things I have to be grateful for. That's why I've sprinkled them across the pages of this book. If you find a few that speak to you, copy them, and tape them up on your bathroom mirror, fridge, or anywhere else you'll see and read them often. Because the thing about being positive is that it can be a self-perpetuating phenomenon. The more upbeat you are, the better you'll feel.

So I guess all this is to say that this book is here to help you feel like the brilliant painter of your own masterpiece, the exciting writer of your own script, the director of your own captivating movie. You're the star of your own show, and you should look like it!

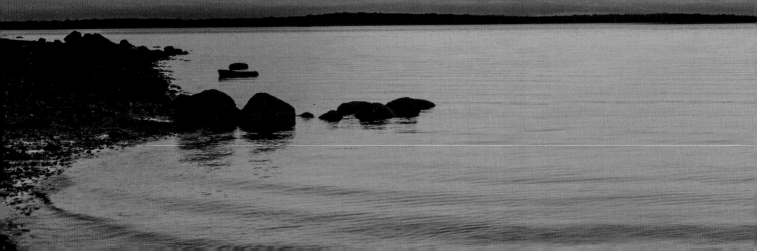

Everything in your life is a reflection of a choice you have made. If you want a different result, make a different choice. Making the healthy choices laid out in this book is a natural part of your vibrant lifestyle, and it will make you feel great and look sensational.

**You're a star—
GO SHINE!**

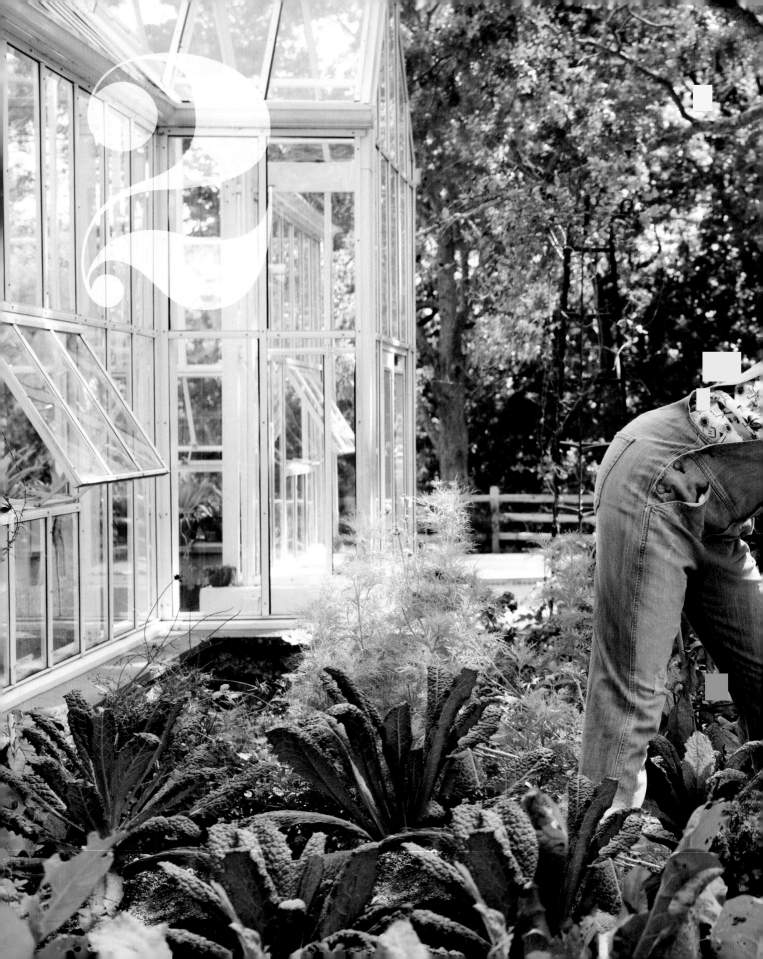

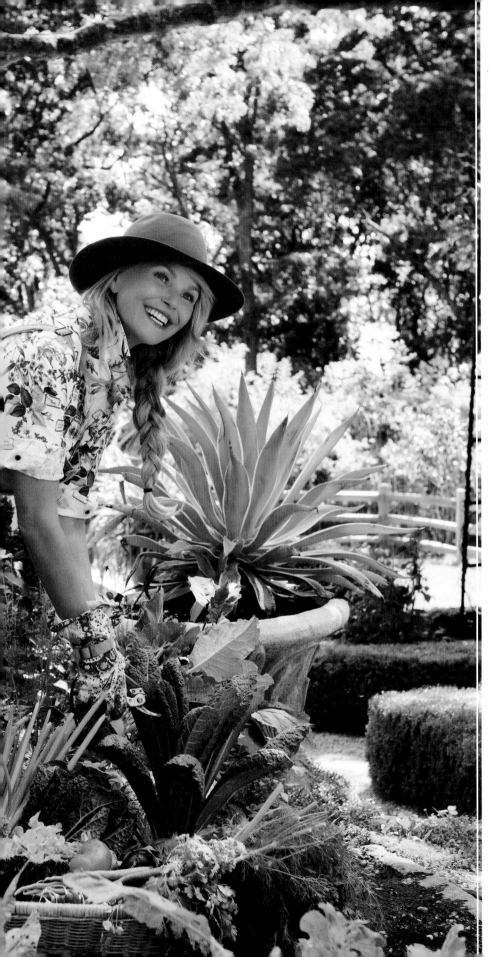

ENLIGHTENED EATING

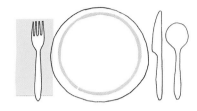

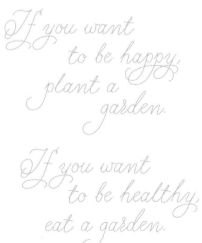

If you want to be happy, plant a garden.

If you want to be healthy, eat a garden.

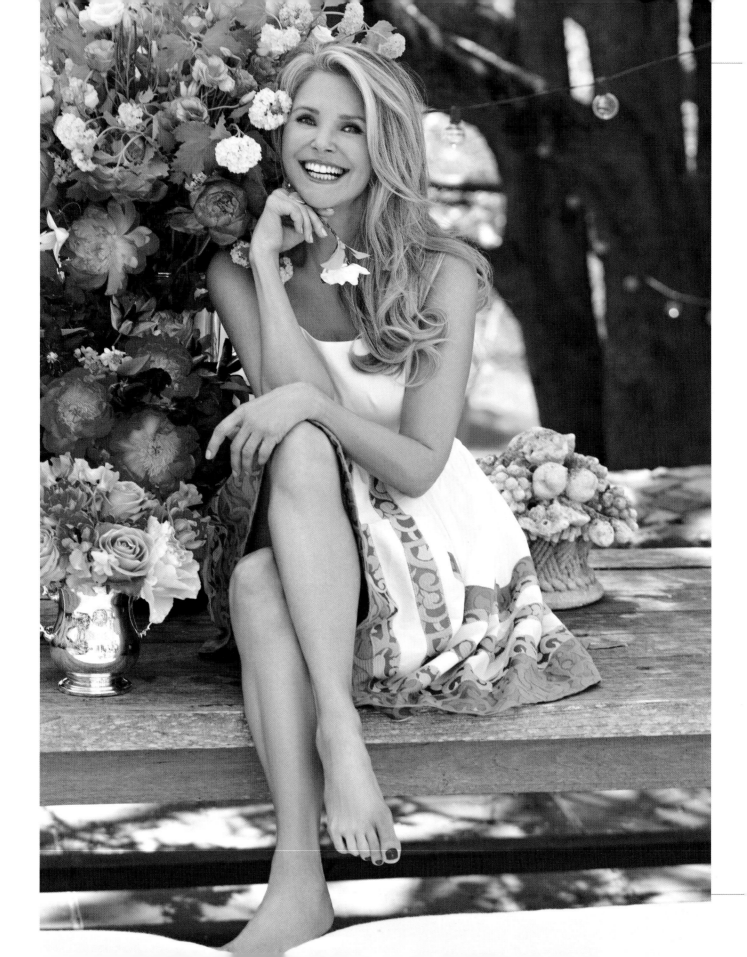

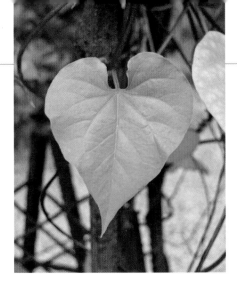

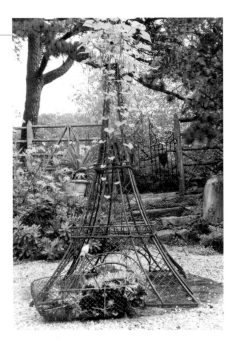

Eating is something we are all pretty good at already, but I'd like to give you some more food for thought—or more precisely, a different way to think about food. I want to help you discover the power of food to fuel your health, your beauty, and your adventures. It's an approach that I like to call enlightened eating (that may also make you lighter too!). In this chapter, I am going to show you the power of healthy food and positive thinking, a combination that will result in a healthier lifestyle. You will feel—and see—the benefits faster than you can say "lacto-ovo-pescatarian vegetarian" (which is the kind of vegetarian I have been for most of my life).

Let me tell you how I came around to eating the way I do. When I was twelve years old, I was leafing through a book on my parents' nightstand, Norman Mailer's novel *Miami and the Siege of Chicago*. It fell open to a page with a graphic description of how animals are treated and killed in Chicago's slaughterhouses, and what I read changed my life forever. I was so horrified that I decided then and there that I did not want to be part of a system that did that to animals. And I never touched another piece of meat again! In a nice touch of karma, I have been reaping the health benefits of that decision ever since.

I didn't know it then, but my decision to stop eating meat has kept me from ingesting fats, antibiotics, and hormones that my body didn't need. What I did understand was that I had to replace the protein I had been getting from meat with other sources. So I started reading up on how to get the nutrients I needed to stay healthy and feel energized. To my delight, I discovered so many delicious ways to get plant-based proteins into my diet. And it brought a new awareness to my health on so many different levels that I had never considered before. I truly believe that decision so many years ago has allowed me to have a forty-plus-year modeling career! I think whether you give up meat entirely or just make a point of eating more plant foods, you will see and feel the rejuvenating results too!

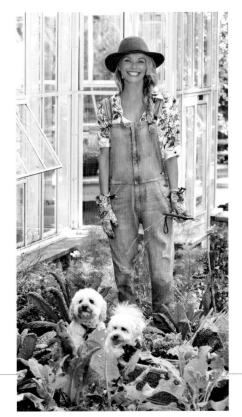

In many cultures, meat represents a much smaller part of the diet than it does in our fast-food culture. Think about it—in Mexico and Cuba and most of the Caribbean, it's rice and beans. In Morocco, it's couscous and garbanzo beans. In Japan, they eat soybeans, tofu, and rice. In India, it's lentils and rice. In Italy, they opt for pasta and vegetables and just small portions of meat. Sounds delicious, doesn't it? This global gourmet menu should be yours too! I also believe that skipping meat—or at least cutting down on your consumption—is a better choice for the planet as well as for your health. A study published in August 2014 in the *Proceedings of the National Academy of Sciences* reported that giving up beef reduces your carbon footprint more than giving up your car.

Do you know where your food has been?

Eating has gotten tricky these days. Events such as the devastating BP oil rig disaster in the Gulf of Mexico, where the Gulf was polluted with both oil and toxic dispersants (which had been banned in England for cancer-causing effects), as well as the ongoing nuclear disaster in Japan that is pouring radioactive isotopes into the Pacific Ocean (which have shown up in kelp in California), have caused me to rethink the safety of consuming fish and most kelp. (I have found a source called **Maine Coast Sea Vegetables** for organic sea vegetables that are chemical-free; they run stringent tests for everything from heavy metals to fertilizer, herbicides, and fuel oil.) Even prior to these events, the public was cautioned against consuming many of the larger species of fish, such as tuna and swordfish, due to contamination from heavy metals like mercury.

Another thing I find alarming is the increasing prevalence of genetically modified organisms (GMOs). This technology involves taking genes from one food and inserting them into another. The idea behind this sort of genetic engineering is to create foods that are more nutritious and plants that are more resistant to drought and other hazards. Sounds great, except for the fact that

we, as consumers of this food, are all forced to be unwitting guinea pigs for big agriculture companies' experiments. And because there are still no laws mandating the labeling of foods containing GMOs, it's impossible to know what you're really eating. An estimated 60 to 70 percent of all processed foods contain GMOs, but you won't find that information anywhere on the ingredients label.

Avoiding genetically modified foods is just one of the many reasons I try to buy and eat organic food as much as possible. It's the best way to avoid as many toxins and impurities in your food as you can. Organic fruits and vegetables aren't treated with pesticides, so you know you aren't consuming potentially harmful chemicals along with your produce. I know that organic options can sometimes be harder to find and are often more expensive. But there are ways to make organic more affordable. Shop only for the produce that's in season (you can even stock up and freeze things like organic berries). Frozen organic vegetables are less expensive than fresh and are available all year round, and they are often mentioned as being more vitamin rich because they are frozen fresh at the source. Consider that over a billion tons of pesticides are used in

the United States every year. The first pesticide to be widely used was DDT, and it took scientists twenty years to figure out that it was harming us! Twenty years from now, what will they be telling us about what they are dumping on our crops today? That's one mystery I won't expose my family to.

Since we are what we eat, shouldn't we know what we're eating?

FOOD FOR THOUGHT

Every year, the **Environmental Working Group** (ewg.org) puts out a *Shopper's Guide to Pesticides in Produce* that features a list of the so-called "Dirty Dozen"—the conventionally grown fruits and vegetables that harbor the most pesticide residue. If nothing else, I always try to eat only organic versions of these foods, and I encourage you to do the same (again, try to find these in season as they will be less expensive, or skip them if you can't get organic). The worst offenders vary from year to year, but apples, strawberries, grapes, celery, peaches, and spinach routinely rank at the top of the list.

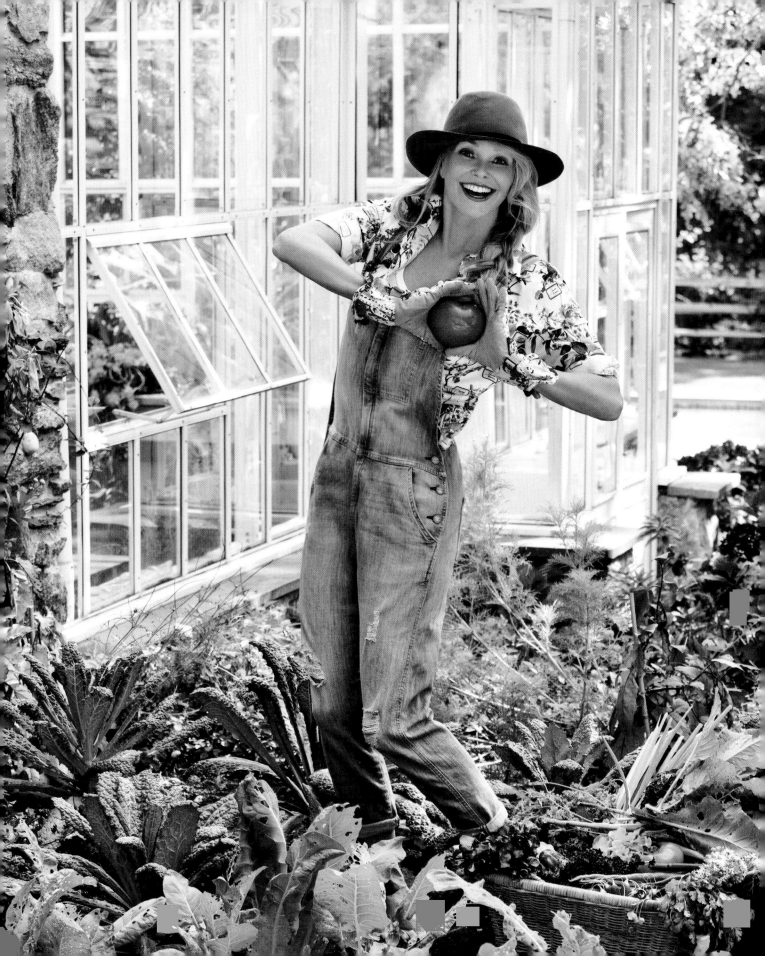

No more "deny-iting"

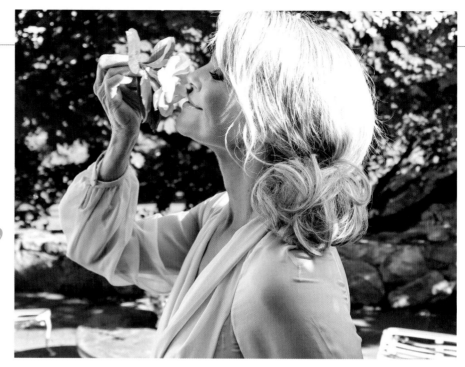

I absolutely LOVE to eat, and the last thing I ever want to do is deny myself delicious food. That is why I'm adamantly opposed to what I call "deny-iting." We've all been there. The second you say, "I'm on a diet," food is the ONLY thing you can think about. And naturally your mind goes right to the foods you *can't* eat, and then you feel like you are denying yourself. This kind of deny dieting, or "deny-iting," will work, but only for a brief period. There's only so long you can suffer deprivation before you give in and binge eat out of anger and frustration, and gain all your weight back. The key to stopping this vicious cycle isn't just changing the way you eat; it's about changing the way you THINK!

So stop searching for whatever trendy diet you think might make you lose weight. Everything you need to lose weight and keep it off is in your head. Accessing the healthiest, most beautiful you is as easy as flipping a switch. You need to focus the spotlight on how you FEEL, not just on how you LOOK (looking great is just a fabulous bonus). My approach to food is not about a quick fix—it's a lifestyle change. And I know that for you to adopt this lifestyle for the long run, it has to be fun, flexible, forgiving, delicious, nutritious, interesting,

family friendly, all-inclusive, easy, and REWARDING!

So let's just agree that you are never "deny-iting" again! Never! Because when you stop thinking about what you CAN'T have (and lamenting it) and start thinking about what you CAN have that will fuel your body, that's when you'll be successful in maintaining your perfect weight and good health. By mindfully making informed choices, you will be rewarded with more energy, a clear, glowing complexion, shinier hair, a trimmer figure, and even see some aches and pains diminish thanks to the amazing healing and protective powers of healthy food.

Ready? Let's start with the simple concept of looking at each bite you take as a golden opportunity—an opportunity to gift yourself with energy and good health. It's all about making the choice to eat the foods that will make you stronger, heal and invigorate you, and keep you running through your busy day. When you think about how valuable each bite can be, you'll never want to DENY your body that advantage. Thinking about

food as a real health and beauty opportunity puts you in control. You can be either a friend to yourself or your own worst enemy. Remember that the difference between who you are and who you want to be is determined by the choices you make. My dad, a writer, always used to say, "You write your own script." The food you write into your script will determine your story line. So for a long, healthy life full of adventures and a storybook ending, start eating the right way right now.

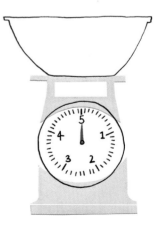

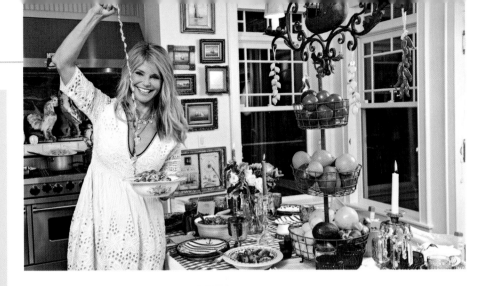

THE BEAUTY OF BEING FLEXIBLE

These days, I eat a mostly vegan diet (no meat or fish, and the only dairy I eat is sheep's- or goat's-milk yogurt), but if I happen to find myself in Italy, then I will make an exception for mozzarella (and maybe even a scoop of gelato). Because I also want to live *la dolce vita*. My point is, you should be able to be flexible and enjoy life and not beat yourself up. Because that enjoyment translates to BEAUTY! I do not believe in missing out, or in feeling guilty for indulging on occasion. Life is a delicious banquet, so gobble it up with gusto. Stick with me, and you will see that JOY is a very important ingredient in my recipe for vibrant health and true beauty.

PRODUCT RAVE

Basta with the "Can't Eat Pasta" routine! Sure you can! When you choose the right pasta, you can eat it every day if you want (I know your kids will). The favorites in my house are **Ancient Harvest Gluten-Free Quinoa Supergrain Pasta** and **truRoots Ancient Grain Pastas** made from organic brown rice, quinoa, amaranth, and corn.

INNER BEAUTY TIP

As consumers, we have the power to affect change in the food industry. The more we all support organic farmers by buying local produce, meat, and dairy, the more prices will come down. The more people who lobby their local supermarkets to include or expand their organic sections, the more options we'll all have to eat well. And the more people who demand transparency in food labeling, the more big corporations will feel the pressure to stop using GMOs—or at least acknowledge using them. (See chapter 9 for organizations that are committed to these causes.) When it comes to protecting our planet and its four-legged inhabitants, check out the **Natural Resources Defense Council** (nrdc.org).

QUICK TIP
KEEP YOUR EYE ON THE PRIZE

Before you prepare a meal or grab a snack, take a few moments to remind yourself of your goals. What's inspiring you to change your routine? Do you want to lose pounds and inches? Are you looking for more energy? To reduce inflammation? To fit into that dress? To lower your cholesterol? To grow old in good health and remain independent? Taking a moment to ask yourself the right questions at the right moment can redirect your willpower and help keep you on the right path.

PRODUCT RAVE

I love **Bio-K probiotics**. I mix them into my sheep's- or goat's-milk yogurt (the one dairy product I do eat regularly) every morning. I credit them with helping keep my immune system strong. Try adding them to whatever type of yogurt you enjoy, or mix them into a smoothie, and you'll see the difference too!

Stocking your enlightened kitchen

Did you know that blueberries and leafy greens make your eyes sparkle? Or that tomatoes have lycopene, which is antiaging? How about walnuts? They are powerhouses full of omega-3s, which smooth skin and add shine to your hair. Kiwis are packed with vitamin C, which prevents wrinkles. (I'll take a case of kiwis, please!) Did you know that the antioxidants in dark chocolate protect skin from sun damage? (I wonder how much we have to eat for that to work. I volunteer for that research project!) My point is that food is incredibly potent, and eating the right food allows you to harness that power.

Stocking your home with power foods is fun. When it comes to food—just as in the rest of my life—I love variety and color! I try to eat a whole cornucopia of different foods to ensure that I'm getting as wide a range of nutrients as possible. But certain things seem to show up on my table more often than others. Here are several foods I can't live without:

KALE

Researchers have identified forty-five different flavonoids in kale, which help account for its antioxidant and anti-inflammatory benefits. I was a fan of kale long before it became the trendy vegetable it is today! I mix it into salads, smoothies, and soups, use it as a pizza topping—it pretty much shows up in at least one meal a day at my house. And the more I hear about it, the more of it I want to eat (same goes for other dark, leafy greens like spinach, collard greens, and arugula).

BROCCOLI

I think I fed my kids broccoli nearly every day when they were growing up, and we all still love it. Like kale, it's chock-full of antioxidants that help prevent cancer and fight inflammation.

BLUEBERRIES

These little blue powerhouses contain antioxidants that may help prevent cancer while improving memory and maintaining eye health.

FLAX AND CHIA SEEDS, WALNUTS, ALMONDS, BRAZIL NUTS

When I stopped eating fish, I increased my intake of these seeds and nuts in order to get a healthy dose of omega-3s—and extra protein—into my diet. I toss them onto yogurt, cereal, or salads, or grind them up and mix them into smoothies.

AVOCADOS

They get a bad rap for being high in fat, but we need some fat in our diet—especially the healthy kind found in avocados. And if you regularly add them to your diet, they may even help eliminate love handles and muffin tops. They contain glutathione, monounsaturated fats, and fiber, which help block intestinal absorption of some types of bad fats (because the place is already taken by the good ones). And because of their high fat content, they're naturally creamy and filling when you blend them into smoothies, spreads, or soups. And of course the eternal favorite, guacamole! OLÉ!

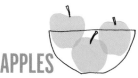

APPLES

I eat one every day. Fujis are my jam! Apples are packed with polyphenols that can help regulate blood sugar and lower cholesterol levels (which can reduce your risk of heart disease). There's even some evidence that eating one before a workout can extend your endurance. No wonder doctors think they're bad for business!

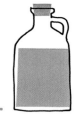

OLIVE OIL

I cook with it, but I also drizzle it onto food after cooking (it adds great flavor). You get the most flavor—and most health benefits—by using darker green, cold-pressed, extra-virgin olive oil.

KIWIS

They have even more vitamin C than an orange and can protect your eyes from macular degeneration. The antioxidants in them are so powerful they may even prevent the DNA damage (and wrinkles) caused by free radicals!

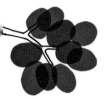

RED & PURPLE GRAPES

Both contain the antioxidant resveratrol, which helps protect against heart disease. You'll get some in wine too (which is more fun—cheers!).

CABBAGE

Part of the cruciferous family of vegetables, cabbage is packed with antioxidants called glucosinolates that have proven cancer-preventing benefits. Red, green, and savoy cabbages provide different patterns of glucosinolates, so eat a whole variety of this wonderfully crunchy vegetable.

PICKLES

Fermented foods are all the rage—pickles, pickled cabbage (like kimchi), fermented tea (kombucha). That's because they are excellent sources of probiotics, the good bacteria that help keep your digestive system healthy and boost your immunity.

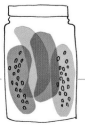

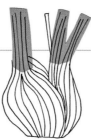

FENNEL

I love eating sautéed fennel or adding it raw to salad for a spicy crunch. And when I do, I'm getting a healthy dose of vitamin C, fiber, folate, and potassium.

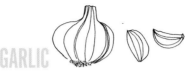

GARLIC

This delicious herb adds such great flavor to everything—plus, it contains unique sulfur compounds that may help improve metabolism, reduce inflammation, and fight infections.

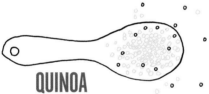

QUINOA

This incredibly nutrient-dense grain is a staple at my house—at lunch, dinner, even breakfast. It is a rich source of fiber, antioxidant phytonutrients, and heart-healthy fats (like oleic acid and omega-3s), but unlike other grains, it's also packed with protein and all nine essential amino acids (great news for vegetarians).

STEEL-CUT OATS

They help lower cholesterol and keep your heart healthy. So I cook up three days' worth at a time, keep them in the fridge, and reheat for a quick, healthy breakfast.

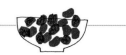

DRIED TART CHERRIES

A handful of these is a yummy snack that's also packed with health benefits. There's evidence that they can help reduce belly fat, reduce muscle soreness after a workout, and even help you get a better night's sleep (they contain the sleep-inducing hormone melatonin).

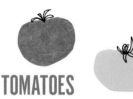

TOMATOES

Raw or cooked, tomatoes are just packed with antioxidants. But their superstar nutrient, lycopene, is most plentiful in cooked red tomatoes. Lycopene has been linked to bone health and a reduced risk of prostate, breast, pancreatic, and lung cancers. And new research has found that a compound in green tomatoes can help you build more muscle.

DARK CHOCOLATE

The flavonols in dark chocolate can help lower blood pressure and improve blood flow to your brain and your heart. Plus, it's the perfect way to satisfy a sweet tooth.

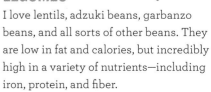

LEGUMES

I love lentils, adzuki beans, garbanzo beans, and all sorts of other beans. They are low in fat and calories, but incredibly high in a variety of nutrients—including iron, protein, and fiber.

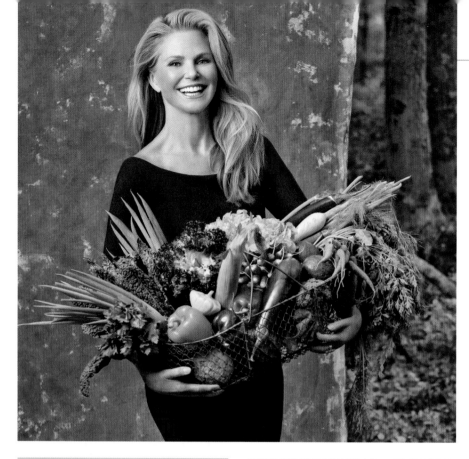

Enlightened snacking

Yummy snacks are definitely not off-limits in my plan! (No "deny-iting," remember?) In fact, I encourage you to use your snacks as yet another opportunity to choose powerful, good-for-you foods. The key to successful snacking (that doesn't turn into overindulging) is portion control. Not an exciting concept, I know, but if you make a real effort to keep the size of your snacks in check, you can indulge daily, without guilt.

EAT THE RAINBOW

For as long as I can remember, I've made a point of including as many different colors as I can in every meal—when my kids were little we called it "eating the rainbow." It's the best way to guarantee that you're getting a wide range of nutrients. And every day, science is proving my theory right. Researchers have identified numerous beneficial antioxidants and phytonutrients in all the colors of fruits and vegetables. Having all those different colors in your diet gives you an array of protection from inflammation and various diseases, including cancer and Alzheimer's.

PRODUCT RAVE

Living Intentions Salad Boosters are such an easy way to add some nutritional *oomph*, not just to salads, but also to cereal, yogurt, soup, anything! The blend includes a mix of pumpkin, sunflower, and chia seeds, spirulina, kelp, and Himalayan crystal salt.

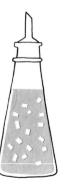

TIME TO
MULTI-TASKERCISE!

Reading, watching TV, or any activity while sitting in a chair doesn't have to be a sedentary activity. To tighten and tone your abs as you read this chapter, try to pull your ribs in flat, visualize trying to hold your waist in, making it as tiny as possible, and feel the deep muscles in your abs working. Keep breathing, keep reading, keep holding and adjusting tighter...it works. And remember, a tight tummy protects your back. You can add on any of the following while keeping your abs tight:

1. Alternate lifting one foot off the ground, then the other.
2. If you have room, extend your leg as you lift.
3. Bend both knees and lift up in this position, round your back, and straighten.

Here are some of my favorites to munch on:

An apple spread with peanut or almond butter

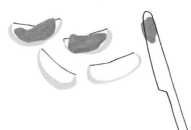

A square of dark chocolate along with a few nuts, dried cranberries, raisins, or açai berries

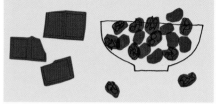

Frozen bananas, grapes, or blueberries

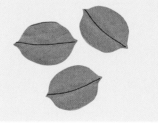

Blend any or all of these fruits and it tastes like you're indulging in ice cream! Use coconut water, orange juice, or Cheribundi juice to help blend—each gives different flavors and delivers a rainbow of nutrition.

A date with a handful of walnuts

Nibbled together, they taste sooo delish!

Baked kale chips sprinkled with salt

Himalayan pink salt is my favorite!

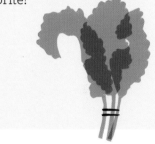

Roasted pumpkin seeds with Himalayan pink salt or sea salt

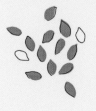

Fresh-cut fennel

Raw or roasted with a little olive oil and a touch of salt

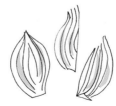

Steamed artichokes

These are great if you're a nibbler—work on one while you watch TV and it'll keep you busy for a long time! Dip the leaves into veggie mayo or oil-and-vinegar dressing.

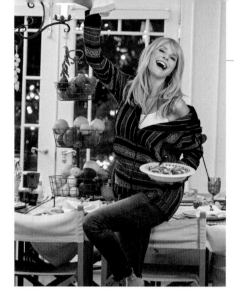

Let's get cooking!

Now that your kitchen is stocked, Chef Gabi is here to show you how to turn these healthy ingredients into delicious meals. Gabriela Monteiro, who has been helping my family eat well for the past four years, is living proof that healthy food never has to be bland or boring! She fills our home daily with mouth-watering aromas of something special in the oven or on the stove, along with plenty of warm smiles and Brazilian music (my fave too!), and she often cooks while we cheer on her Brazilian soccer team (unless they are playing the United States!).

Gabi knows how to make every meal a celebration of wonderful tastes—that also just so happen to be extremely nutritious and good for you! She has introduced me to so many new and delicious dishes, has shown me how to make my old healthy recipes tastier, and has taught me tricks for eating well even when time is limited. She and I definitely share a love affair with food (she's just way more talented than I am when it comes to preparing it).

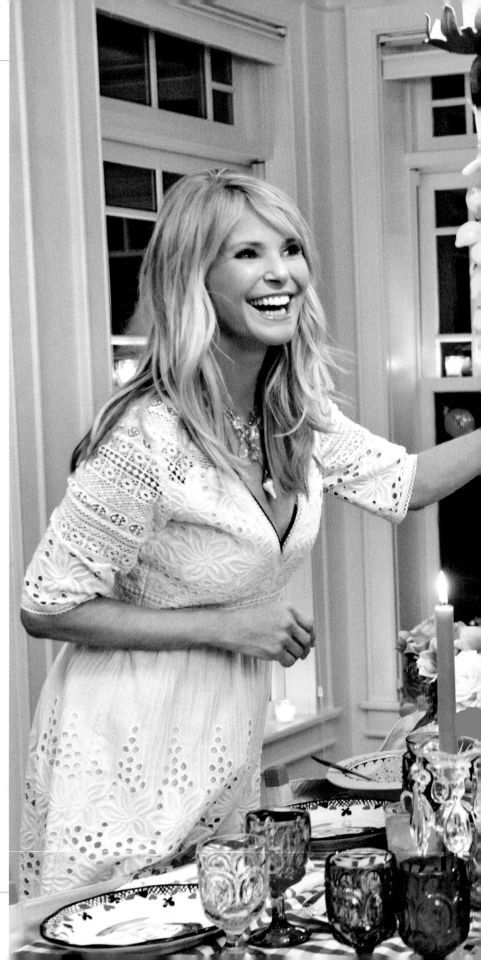

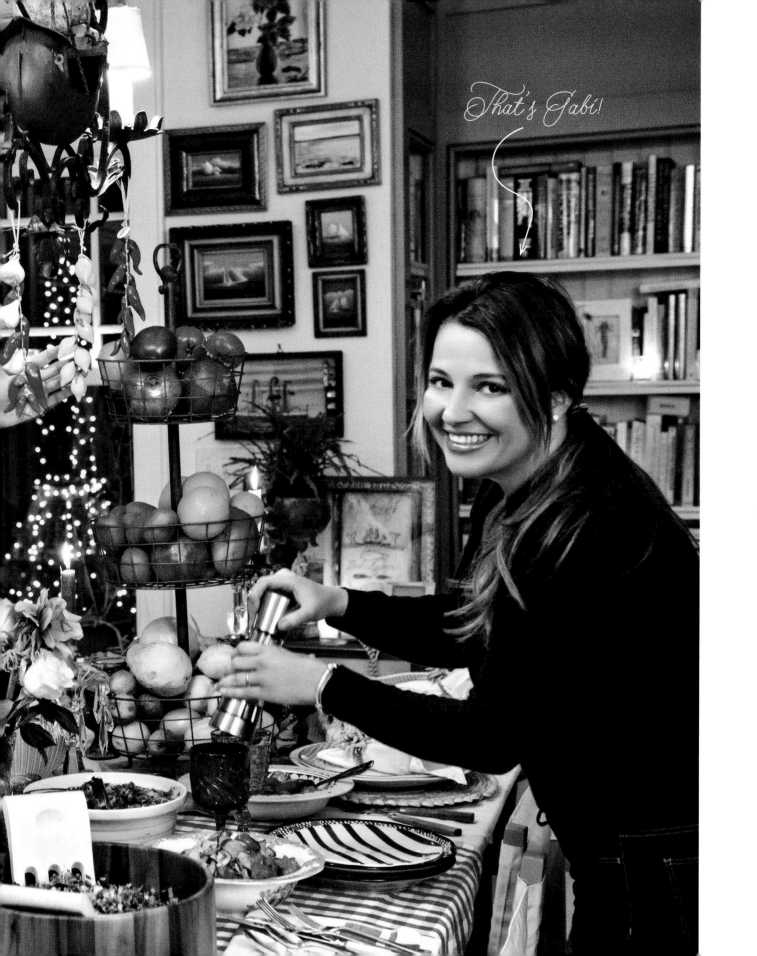

That's Gabi!

My favorite recipes

I know that not everyone is lucky enough to have a Gabi in their kitchen, so I've asked her to share some of our favorite recipes that are simple enough for anyone to prepare—even on the busiest days!

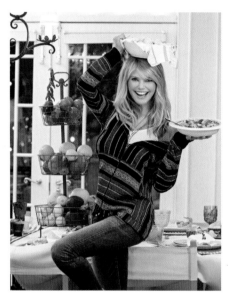

QUICK TIP
COOK FASTER

I used to be afraid of pressure cookers, but they are a MUST for saving time.

Gabi uses a pressure cooker several times a week to shave valuable time off dinner prep. A pressure cooker can cook food—like beans, potatoes, and even meat—up to 70 percent faster than doing it on the stove.

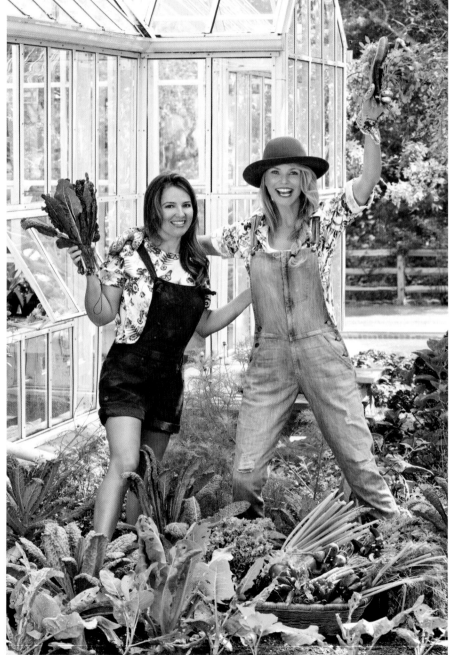

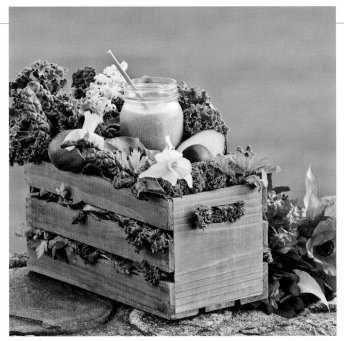

Green Smoothie

I drink this delicious concoction almost every day. Instead of grabbing a coffee to fight the afternoon energy slump, I use this to perk me up.

SERVES 1

1 cup chopped fresh kale
¼ avocado
Juice of 1 orange
Juice of ½ lime
1 cup ice
½ cup coconut water

Combine all the ingredients in a blender and blend for about 2 minutes, until smooth. Serve right away. And feel free to get creative with this basic recipe (adding kiwis, cucumbers, or other vegetables or fruit depending on what you have on hand).

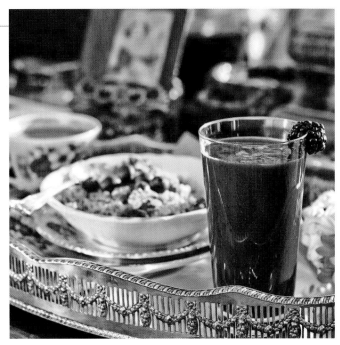

Açai, Banana, and Berries Smoothie

This smoothie gives you a major antioxidant boost, thanks to the variety of berries. Plus it's so delicious it almost feels like dessert!

SERVES 1

½ banana
½ cup fresh raspberries
½ cup fresh blackberries
½ cup ice
½ cup water or apple juice
1 frozen smoothie pack açai puree (100 grams)
Fresh mint or berries for garnish (optional)

Combine all the ingredients in a blender and blend for about 2 minutes, until smooth.

Garnish with fresh mint or berries, if desired, and serve right away.

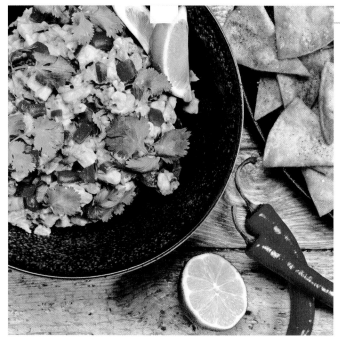
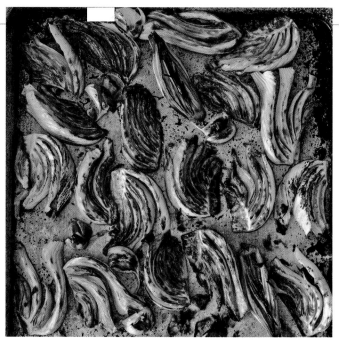

Guacamole

Avocados are rich in the good kinds of fat, so as long as you skip greasy chips in favor of healthier dipping alternatives, you can indulge in guacamole without guilt.

SERVES 4

2 avocados
1 garlic clove, minced
2 jalapeños, seeded and chopped
¼ cup coarsely chopped fresh cilantro, plus more for garnish
1 medium tomato, diced
Juice of 1 lime
Salt and freshly ground black pepper
Lime wedges, for garnish
Healthy chips, for serving

In a medium bowl, smash the avocados with a fork. Add the remaining ingredients and gently mix it all together. Garnish with some fresh cilantro and a few wedges of lime.

Serve with healthy chips like quinoa or bean chips (just watch out for their sodium levels).

Roasted Fennel

Fennel has a unique, almost licorice-like taste, and when you roast it, that flavor mellows into something incredibly delicious.

SERVES 6

4 large fennel bulbs
¼ cup extra-virgin olive oil
½ teaspoon sea salt
¼ teaspoon freshly ground black pepper

Preheat the oven to 400°F.

Remove the stems from the fennel, reserving a few fronds for garnish, and halve the bulbs lengthwise. With the cut side down, slice the bulbs into about 1/2-inch-thick slices. Spread the fennel slices on a baking sheet, coat with the olive oil, salt, and pepper, and toss with your hands. Roast the fennel slices for about 1 hour, turning them once after 30 minutes, making sure they get cooked evenly. Once they are golden brown and crispy, remove from the oven and garnish with the reserved fennel fronds.

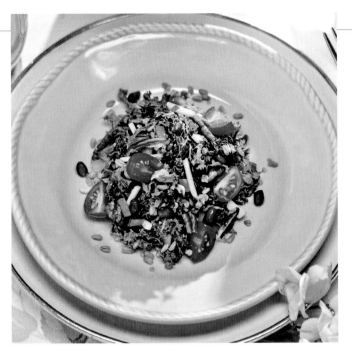

Chopped Kale Salad

I eat some variation of this salad nearly every day. You can add in different veggies or grains or sprinkle in some dried cranberries or dried cherries, or vary the nuts and seeds to add color and more nutrients.

SERVES 6

4 cups organic kale leaves
Seeds from ¼ pomegranate
½ yellow bell pepper, diced
½ orange bell pepper, diced
1 cup diced cherry tomatoes
1 cup cooked barley
Handful of chopped pecans, toasted
½ Granny Smith apple, julienned
½ cup Honey Vinaigrette (recipe follows)

Rinse kale leaves and dry them in a salad spinner. Chop the kale into 1/2- to 1-inch strips and place in a large bowl. Add the pomegranate seeds, bell peppers, tomatoes, barley, pecans, and apple and toss to combine.

Drizzle the *Honey Vinaigrette* over the salad and serve.

Honey Vinaigrette

MAKES ²/₃ CUP

Zest and juice of 1 lemon
1 tablespoon honey (preferably local honey)
1 tablespoon white balsamic vinegar
1 tablespoon rice vinegar
Pinch of cayenne pepper
⅓ cup extra-virgin olive oil

In a small bowl, whisk together the lemon zest and juice, honey, vinegars, and cayenne. While whisking, slowly stream in the olive oil until emulsified.

Brussels Sprout Fall Salad

I try to eat seasonally, so when Brussels sprouts show up at my local farmer's market, I come up with as many ways to eat them as I can. Adding nuts and seeds gives this salad great crunch and a boost of nutrients.

SERVES 4

4 cups Brussels sprout leaves, lightly blanched
¼ cup dried cranberries
¼ cup nuts, such as macadamia, pecans, or roasted hazelnuts, coarsely chopped
Handful of pumpkin seeds (pepitas), toasted
1 carrot, sliced paper-thin on a mandoline
1 avocado, diced
⅓ cup Citrus-Almond Vinaigrette (recipe follows)

Dry the Brussels sprout leaves very well in a salad spinner.

In a bowl, combine the Brussels sprout leaves, cranberries, nuts, pumpkin seeds, carrot, and diced avocado.

Pour the ***Citrus-Almond Vinaigrette*** over the salad and mix it gently.

Citrus-Almond Vinaigrette

MAKES ABOUT ⅓ CUP

2 tablespoons extra-virgin olive oil
1 tablespoon almond oil
1 teaspoon honey or light agave syrup
1 tablespoon apple cider vinegar
¼ teaspoon salt
½ teaspoon fresh lemon juice

In a small bowl, whisk together all the ingredients.

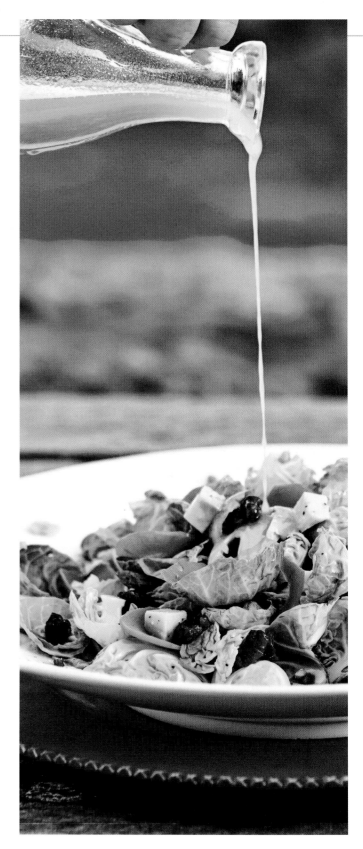

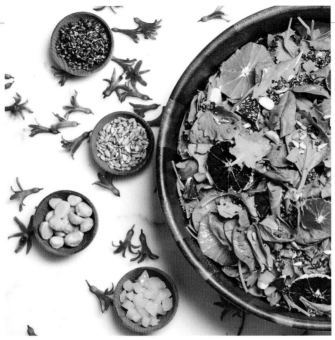

Baby Kale Salad

This is another variation on my favorite Chopped Kale Salad (page 39). Because this salad also boasts quinoa and toasted walnuts, it's not just a beautifying, health-rendering, delish delight, but it also provides protein to power you through your afternoon!

SERVES 4

4 cups organic baby kale
1 yellow bell pepper, diced
½ cup cooked red quinoa (see note)
Handful of chopped walnuts, toasted
⅓ cup Balsamic Vinaigrette (recipe follows)
2 sliced blood oranges to garnish

Rinse the kale and dry in a salad spinner. Chop the kale into 1- to 2-inch strips and place them in a large bowl. Add the bell pepper, quinoa, and walnuts and toss to combine.

Drizzle the *Balsamic Vinaigrette* over the salad and serve.

Note: To cook quinoa, use a ratio of 2 cups water to 1 cup quinoa. Bring the water to a boil, then add the quinoa, reduce the heat to low, cover, and cook for 10 to 15 minutes.

Balsamic Vinaigrette

MAKES ABOUT 1 CUP

2 tablespoons minced shallots
¼ cup balsamic vinegar
1 teaspoon whole grain mustard
Pinch of salt
Pinch of freshly ground black pepper
½ cup extra-virgin olive oil

In a small bowl, mix the shallots, vinegar, mustard, salt, and pepper. Slowly add the olive oil, and whisk together with the other ingredients.

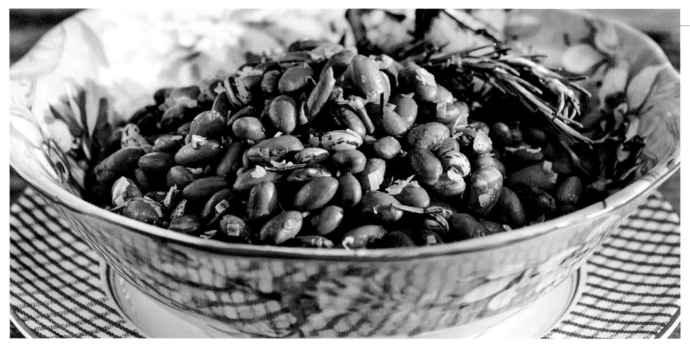

Cranberry Beans

You can find these pink-speckled beans fresh in the late summer and early fall, which is a great time to enjoy their rich, nutty flavor. But if you fall in love with them (as I have!), you can buy them dried all year round.

SERVES 6

1 tablespoon plus 2 teaspoons extra-virgin olive oil
½ cup minced shallots
4 garlic cloves, crushed
2 cups shelled fresh cranberry beans
2 cups vegetable broth
Freshly ground black pepper
2 teaspoons chopped fresh rosemary
2 teaspoons lemon zest
1 tablespoon lemon juice
Pinch of cayenne pepper, or to taste
Salt
1 tablespoon chopped fresh flat-leaf parsley

In a Dutch oven, heat 1 tablespoon of the olive oil over medium heat. Add the shallots and stir for 2 to 3 minutes. Add the garlic and cook for 1 minute. Stir in the beans, vegetable broth, and black pepper. Bring to a boil, reduce the heat to low, cover, and simmer until the beans begin to swell, 20 to 25 minutes. Uncover and continue cooking until the liquid reduces and the beans are tender, 5 to 10 minutes more. Add the rosemary, lemon zest, lemon juice, and cayenne. Season with salt and black pepper. Remove from the heat, stir in the remaining olive oil, and garnish with the parsley.

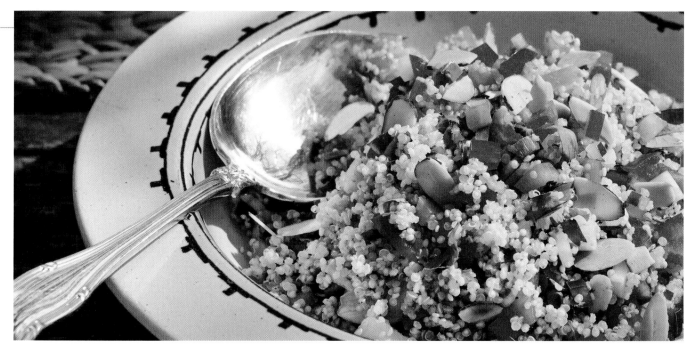

Quinoa Pico de Gallo Salad

Quinoa is called a "super grain" for good reason—it's one of the few nonmeat foods that provide all nine essential amino acids. And have I mentioned, it's also SO delicious?!

SERVES 4

3 cups cooked quinoa (see note, page 41)
1 medium red tomato, diced
1 medium yellow tomato, diced
¼ cup chopped red onion
½ cup diced cucumber
1 cup chopped arugula
¼ cup chopped scallion
½ cup chopped fresh cilantro, plus more for garnish
1 bell pepper, diced
½ cup sliced almonds, toasted
Lemon-Garlic Vinaigrette (recipe follows)
1 jalapeño, seeded and chopped (optional)

In a large bowl, combine all the ingredients except the dressing and the jalapeño. Drizzle the *Lemon-Garlic Vinaigrette* over the salad and gently mix before serving. Garnish with fresh cilantro and chopped jalapeño.

Lemon-Garlic Vinaigrette

MAKES ½ CUP
Juice of 1 lemon
¼ cup extra-virgin olive oil
1 tablespoon red wine vinegar
1 garlic clove, minced
Pinch of red pepper flakes (optional)
Sea salt and freshly ground black pepper

In a small bowl, whisk together all the ingredients.

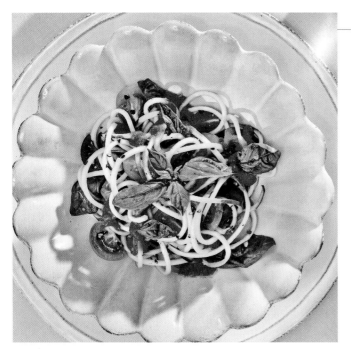

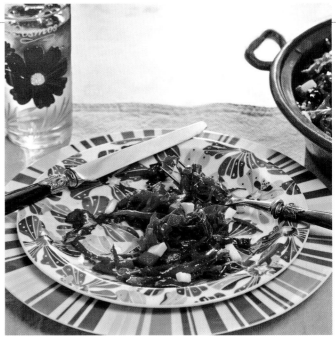

"Zoodles"
with Fresh Tomato Sauce

I absolutely LOVE pasta, but this fresh take replaces the noodles with veggies for a meal that's quick, easy, and oh-so healthy!

SERVES 2

3 medium zucchini
3 tablespoons extra-virgin olive oil
3 garlic cloves, lightly crushed
2 pints cherry tomatoes
Himalayan pink salt and freshly ground black pepper
½ cup fresh basil leaves
Freshly grated pecorino cheese

Use a spiral vegetable slicer to cut the zucchini into noodles. Rinse the "zoodles" with hot water for 30 seconds. Set aside in a large bowl. In a medium saucepan, heat the olive oil and garlic over medium heat. Let the garlic flavor the oil for about 2 minutes (don't let it burn). Remove the garlic and add the tomatoes, salt, and pepper, stirring occasionally. Reduce the heat to medium-low. Add half the fresh basil and cover partially with a lid. Simmer for 15 to 20 minutes, then strain the sauce and pour it over the "zoodles." Serve with pecorino and the remaining fresh basil.

Red Cabbage

Cabbage is a great source of cancer-fighting glucosinolates. I toss it raw into salads for extra crunch, but this cooked version makes an excellent side dish to just about any entrée.

SERVES 4

2 tablespoons Earth Balance vegan spread or extra-virgin olive oil
1 shallot, diced
4 cups shredded red cabbage
1 bay leaf
2 tablespoons chopped fresh parsley, plus more for garnish
½ cup diced green apples
¼ cup apple cider vinegar
3 tablespoons water or vegetable broth
1 teaspoon sea salt
¼ teaspoon freshly ground black pepper
¼ teaspoon freshly grated nutmeg
¼ cup green apple, diced, for garnish

In a medium Dutch oven, melt the vegan spread or heat the oil over medium-high heat, then add the shallot, cabbage, bay leaf, parsley, and apples. Pour in the vinegar and water or vegetable broth and season with the salt, pepper, and nutmeg. Bring to a boil, then reduce the heat to low, cover, and simmer until the cabbage is tender, about 1 hour. Sprinkle with diced green apple and serve.

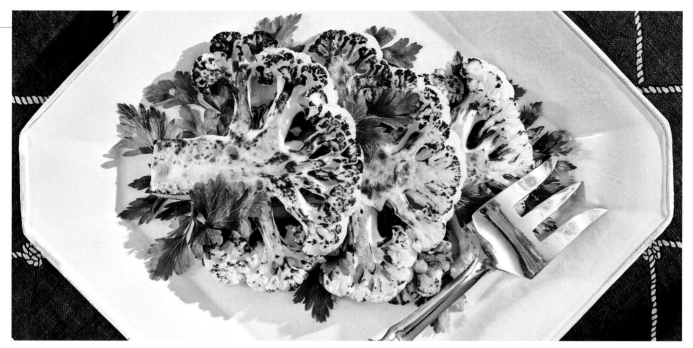

Roasted Cauliflower
with Extra-Virgin Olive Oil and Curry Seasoning

Cooking with fresh herbs and spices not only adds tremendous flavor, but can also add some serious nutrition. Ginger and turmeric are both potent anti-inflammatories, and cumin may have cancer-fighting powers.

SERVES 6

1 large head cauliflower
Salt and freshly ground black pepper
2 tablespoons extra-virgin olive oil
1 teaspoon grated fresh ginger
1 teaspoon ground cumin
½ teaspoon ground turmeric
Small handful of fresh cilantro, chopped, for garnish

Preheat the oven to 400°F.

Trim the stem end of the cauliflower, leaving the core intact. Using a large knife, cut the cauliflower from top to base into three ¾-inch-thick "steaks." (There will be some loose cauliflower pieces—I usually roast them too, or save them for another recipe.) Season each steak with salt and pepper on both sides and arrange them in one layer on a baking sheet.

In a small bowl, whisk together the olive oil, ginger, cumin, and turmeric. Brush or spoon the mixture over the cauliflower steaks.

Roast the cauliflower steaks until tender, about 15 minutes, flipping them halfway through to make sure they get golden brown on both sides. Garnish with cilantro and serve.

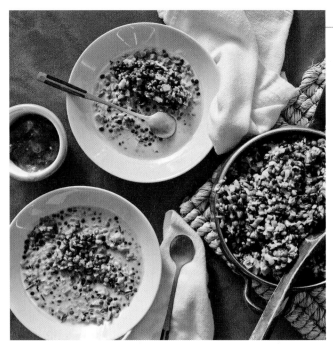

Lentil Curry Stew
with Vegetables

This hearty, meatless stew makes a great meal on a cold, wintry evening. And it's even better left over for lunch the next day!

SERVES 6

1½ cups uncooked lentils, such as red lentils, rinsed
2 tablespoons coconut oil
1 small yellow onion, chopped
2 garlic cloves, minced
2 celery stalks, chopped
2 medium carrots, chopped
1 tablespoon curry powder
½ teaspoon ground coriander
Freshly ground black pepper
¼ cup chopped fresh Italian parsley, plus more
    for garnish
1 cup vegetable broth
⅓ cup unsweetened coconut milk
Pinch of Himalayan pink salt

Place the lentils in a medium saucepan and add water to cover. Bring to a boil and cook the lentils for about 10 minutes, until al dente. Drain the lentils and set aside.

In the same pot, heat the coconut oil, then sauté the onion and garlic for about 4 minutes. Add the celery and carrots and cook for 3 minutes more. Next, add the cooked lentils, curry powder, coriander, pepper, parsley, and vegetable broth. Cover and cook over medium-low heat for 10 minutes. Add the coconut milk and the pink Himalayan salt to taste, and garnish with fresh parsley. Serve warm.

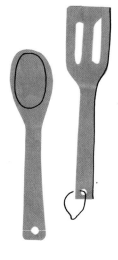

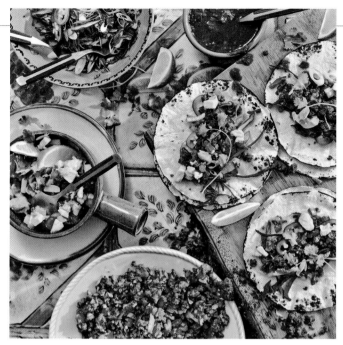

Vegetarian Tacos
with Chipotle Sauce

Mexican food gets a bad rap for being greasy and high in calories. But these tacos, made with fresh, healthy ingredients, are as good for you as they are delicious.

SERVES 2

TACO FILLING
2 tablespoons sunflower oil
½ medium red onion, chopped
2 garlic cloves, chopped
1 cup ground soy
1 large tomato, diced
1 jalapeño, thinly sliced
½ cup chopped fresh cilantro, plus more for garnish
1 teaspoon ground coriander or cumin
Pinch of cayenne pepper
Himalayan pink salt and freshly ground black pepper

AVOCADO SALSA
2 avocados, diced
Juice of 1 lime
2 Roma or heirloom tomatoes, diced
1 cup chopped fresh cilantro
Himalayan pink salt

CHIPOTLE SAUCE
2 Roma tomatoes
2 chipotle chiles from a can of chipotle chiles in adobo
(use more if you want it hotter)
4 sprigs fresh cilantro

CABBAGE SALAD
1 cup shredded red cabbage, plus more for garnish
2 tablespoons chopped scallions, plus more for garnish
½ teaspoon apple cider vinegar
Himalayan pink salt and freshly ground black pepper

TO ASSEMBLE
6 gluten-free corn tortillas   Chopped fresh cilantro
Shredded red cabbage   1 lime, cut into wedges
Chopped scallions

Make the taco filling: Heat the sunflower oil in a medium-sized skillet over medium heat. Sauté the onion and garlic until softened, about 4 minutes. Add the ground soy, tomato, jalapeño, cilantro, coriander, cayenne, salt, and black pepper. Turn the heat to medium-low; stir, and cook for 5 minutes. Remove from the heat, cover with a lid, and set aside.

Make the avocado salsa: In a medium bowl, gently mix the avocado, lime juice, tomatoes, cilantro, and salt. Set aside.

Make the chipotle sauce: Blacken the tomatoes directly on the stove burner, holding them above the flame with a set of metal tongs. It takes about 1 minute to broil each tomato over a burner with the heat set to medium-high. Transfer the tomatoes to a blender and add the chiles, cilantro, and ½ cup water. Pulse three times—do not puree! Transfer the sauce to a bowl and set aside.

Make the cabbage salad: In a medium bowl, mix the cabbage and scallions together, sprinkle with the vinegar, and toss to coat. Add salt and pepper to taste.

Assemble the tacos: Using the stove burner and tongs, char each tortilla over the heat on both sides. Once charred, set each tortilla on a serving platter, top with ¼ cup of the filling, and drizzle with chipotle sauce. Top each with the cabbage salad and serve with the avocado salsa and any remaining chipotle sauce on the side. Garnish with shredded red cabbage, scallions, cilantro, and lime wedges.

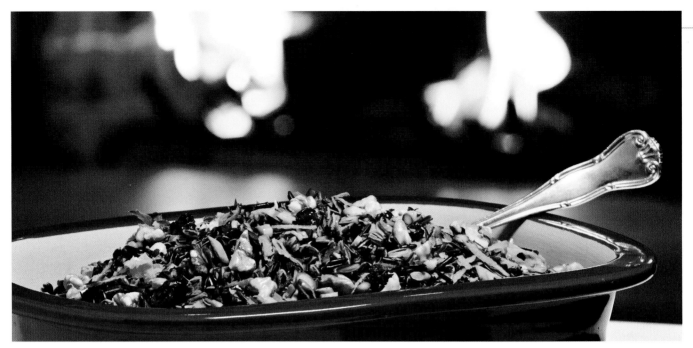

Thanksgiving Rice

Whenever we have this at dinner, I always make enough to leave leftovers. This salad is delicious the next day for lunch—or even breakfast!

SERVES 6

3 cups cooked wild rice
½ cup walnuts, toasted and coarsely chopped
¾ cup dried cranberries, coarsely chopped
½ cup cooked green beans, chopped
½ cup shredded carrots
¼ cup chopped scallions, plus more for garnish
¼ cup fresh flat-leaf parsley leaves, coarsely chopped
½ cup Lemon-Sesame Vinaigrette (recipe follows)
Sea salt and freshly ground black pepper

In a large bowl, combine the rice, walnuts, cranberries, green beans, carrots, scallions, and parsley. Whisk the *Lemon-Sesame Vinaigrette* again, drizzle it over the rice mixture, and toss to combine.

Taste and season with salt and pepper as needed. Garnish with scallion. Serve at room temperature or chilled.

Lemon-Sesame Vinaigrette

MAKES ½ CUP

¼ cup white wine vinegar
3 tablespoons toasted sesame oil
4 teaspoons pomegranate molasses or honey
4 teaspoons finely chopped shallot (from about ½ medium shallot)
1 teaspoon finely grated lemon zest
1 teaspoon sea salt
½ teaspoon freshly ground black pepper

In a small bowl, whisk together all the ingredients until combined.

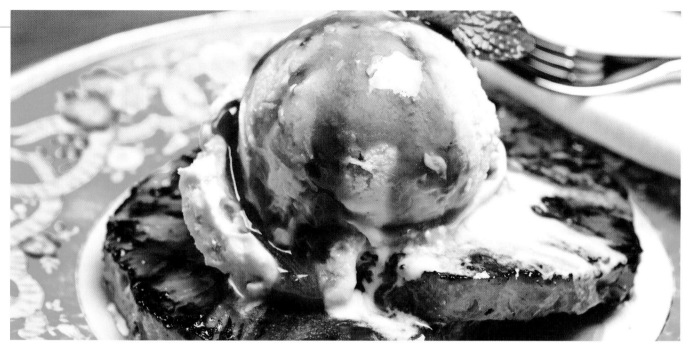

Grilled Pineapple
with Almond Milk Ice Cream and Maple Syrup Glaze

This is one of the fastest and yummiest desserts ever. In the summer, try it with fresh peach halves instead of pineapple.

SERVES 4

3 tablespoons maple syrup
1 teaspoon grated fresh ginger
4 (½-inch-thick) pineapple slices
1 teaspoon coconut oil
Almond or coconut milk ice cream, for serving
Fresh mint, for garnish

In a small bowl, mix the maple syrup and ginger. Brush the mixture over the pineapple slices on both sides. Save the remaining maple mixture.

Heat a grill pan over medium-high heat and brush it with some coconut oil.

Place the pineapple slices on the grill pan and cook for 3 minutes on each side, rotating the slices to get grill marks on both sides.

Serve warm, with almond or coconut milk ice cream. Drizzle some of the remaining maple mixture over the pineapple and ice cream. Garnish with some fresh mint leaves.

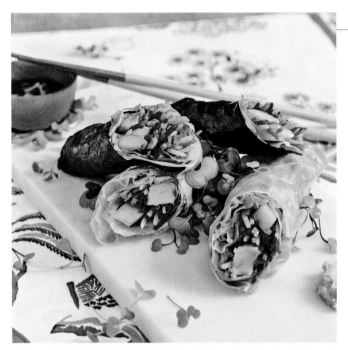

Vegetarian Spring Rolls
with Ponzu Sauce & Wasabi

These are almost as fun to make as they are to eat. Prep the veggies ahead of time and then get the whole family involved in the rolling. You can use all rice paper or nori sheets if you like; we do a mixture of both.

MAKES 35 PIECES

4 sheets rice paper
3 sheets certified organic nori
1 head Boston or butter lettuce
2 medium rainbow carrots, julienned
1 cucumber, cut into ¼-inch strips
1 avocado, cut into ¼-inch strips
½ cup microgreens, plus more for garnish
Ponzu sauce
Coconut aminos
Chopped scallions
Wasabi paste

Brush the rice paper or nori sheets with water until they start to get soft. Clean each leaf of the Boston lettuce and lay one or two leaves over each sheet. Next, add the carrots, cucumber, and avocado, and spread some microgreens on top. Using a sushi mat, roll each sheet slowly until you form it into a roll. Cut rice paper rolls crosswise into 2½-inch pieces and nori rolls into 1½-inch pieces and arrange on a platter. Garnish with the microgreens.

Serve the rolls with ponzu sauce (I add a teaspoon of coconut aminos and some chopped scallions to store-bought ponzu) and wasabi paste on the side.

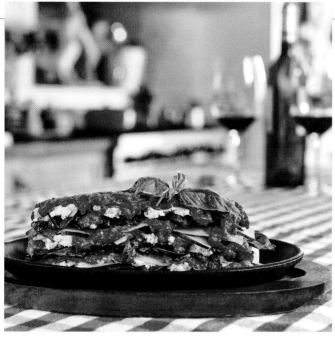

Zucchini Lasagna

Pasta is always a huge hit in our house, so it's no surprise that this lasagna is one of our favorites. It's gluten-free and dairy-free, but I promise, you won't miss either!

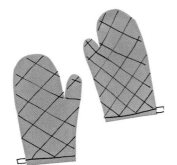

SERVES 4

TOMATO SAUCE
1½ tablespoons extra-virgin olive oil
¼ cup onion, finely chopped
Pinch of red pepper flakes
2 garlic cloves, lightly crushed
10 plum tomatoes, peeled and seeded,
    or 1 (28-ounce) can plum tomatoes
1 teaspoon chopped fresh oregano
1 teaspoon Himalayan pink salt
Freshly ground black pepper
About 10 leaves fresh basil

LASAGNA
4 to 6 gluten-free lasagna noodles
2 medium zucchini, thinly sliced lengthwise with a
    mandoline (using the safety glove)
½ cup shredded mozzarella-style vegetable cheese
1 cup sautéed spinach
2 garlic cloves, chopped
Chopped fresh basil

Preheat the oven to 370°F.

Make the tomato sauce: In a large straight-sided skillet, heat the olive oil over medium heat. Add the onion, red pepper flakes, and garlic. Cook for about 3 minutes.

Add the tomatoes, oregano, salt, pepper, and half the basil. Bring the sauce to a simmer, cover, and cook for 15 to 20 minutes. Remove and discard the garlic cloves.

Make the lasagna: In a large pot of boiling water, cook the gluten-free noodles following the instructions on the package until al dente. Drain.

In an 8 x 8-inch lasagna pan, spread some of the tomato sauce. Arrange 4 to 6 zucchini slices over the sauce. Top with some of the "cheese," spinach, garlic, fresh basil, and a layer of noodles to fit. Continue layering until you are out of ingredients.

Bake the lasagna for 40 to 50 minutes. Garnish with remaining basil before serving.

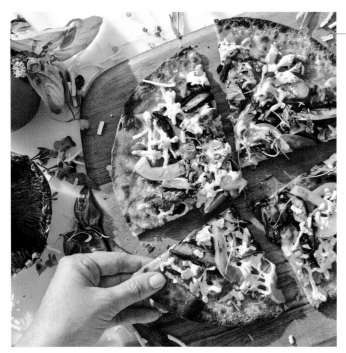

Portobello, Roasted Peppers & Microgreens Pizza

This recipe uses tortillas in place of pizza crust, so it's easy to whip up any time with whatever toppings you have on hand.

SERVES 3

SAUCE
2 medium tomatoes, diced
1 garlic clove
6 fresh basil leaves
Pinch of dried oregano
Salt and freshly ground black pepper
1½ tablespoons extra-virgin olive oil

TOPPINGS
2 portobello mushrooms
1 red bell pepper, seeded and quartered
Salt and freshly ground black pepper
1 cup shredded mozzarella-style vegetable cheese
½ cup microgreens or chopped arugula

CRUST
3 brown rice tortillas
½ tablespoon extra-virgin olive oil

Preheat the oven to 375°F.

Make the sauce: Blend all the ingredients together. Don't blend too long, as the sauce should have a chunky texture.

Prepare the toppings: On a baking sheet greased with olive oil, roast the portobello mushrooms and the bell pepper, seasoned with salt and pepper, for about 10 minutes. Let them cool; slice and reserve. Turn the oven up to 400°F.

Assemble the pizzas: Brush the tortillas with olive oil. Place the tortillas on a baking sheet. Spread some tomato sauce on each tortilla. Add "cheese." Add the roasted portobello mushroom and bell pepper on top of the cheese. Bake for 7 minutes.

Before serving, garnish with some microgreens and drizzle with some olive oil. Cut each into 4 slices and serve warm.

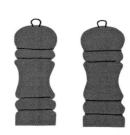

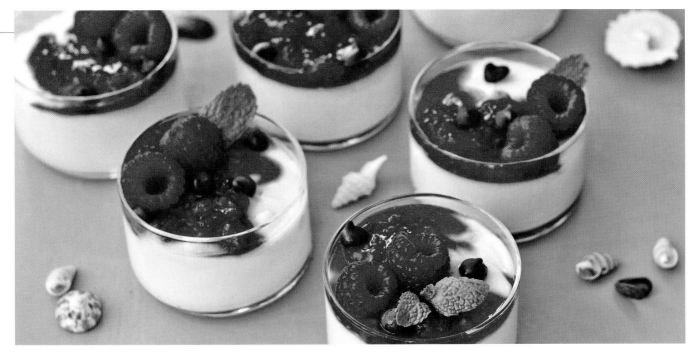

Coconut Pudding
with Maple Sugar, Raspberry Sauce, and Dark Chocolate Chips

Dessert is definitely not off-limits in my healthy eating plan. I just look at it as another opportunity to add more nutrient-packed ingredients (in this case, dark chocolate, berries, maple syrup) into my day.

SERVES 4

2 cups coconut milk
3 tablespoons cornstarch
2 tablespoons maple sugar
½ teaspoon vanilla extract
1 pint fresh raspberries, with a few set aside for garnish
1 tablespoon maple syrup
2 tablespoons dark chocolate chips
Fresh mint, for garnish

In a saucepan, mix the coconut milk, cornstarch, maple sugar, and vanilla. Cook over medium heat, stirring, until the mixture has a pudding consistency. Remove from the heat and let cool for 5 minutes. Transfer the pudding to individual serving dishes. Refrigerate, covered, for about 30 minutes.

Meanwhile, in a small saucepan, combine the raspberries and maple syrup. Cook over low heat, stirring with a wooden spoon and smashing up the raspberries a little bit. Cook for about 2 minutes, or just long enough for the raspberries to release their juices.

Pour some sauce over each pudding and garnish with the dark chocolate chips, whole raspberries, and mint while the sauce is still warm.

4 days of menus

Here is a list of the dishes I ate over a sample four-day period. These foods are all pretty nutrient-packed but still really delicious. Feel free to swap the meals on different days. For the more complicated dishes with more ingredients, I refer you to the page number where you'll find the recipe. Enjoy!

DAY 1

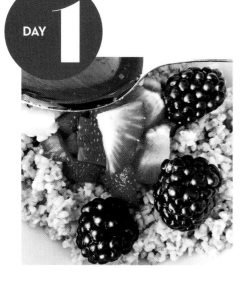

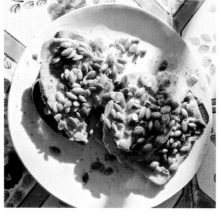

BREAKFAST

Steel-cut oats with strawberries and maple syrup. I make three servings at a time and reheat it the next two days for myself or my daughter Sailor—or both! It saves on cooking time to make a larger batch, and you can even separate and freeze individual portions to microwave when you're really in a hurry!

LUNCH

Timeless avocado sandwich. Savor the flavor, reap the health and beauty benefits. From regulating your BMI to reducing inflammation and cholesterol, this sandwich also helps you absorb your beauty-boosting carotenoids, and it is sooo satisfying! I cut the avocado in half, then hit the seed with the sharp side of my knife to just lift it out. Scoop out the avocado flesh with a spoon and squish it onto a slice of toast. Sometimes I like to drizzle olive oil on the toast (unless I'm trying to slim down after a holiday) and sprinkle lightly with salt and pepper and some seeds to add crunch. This is a versatile lunch I depend on.

DINNER

Chopped salad. Chopped romaine lettuce with grape tomatoes, roasted corn, cucumber, and avocado; and an olive oil, champagne vinegar, and Dijon mustard vinaigrette.

Boiled and smashed new red potatoes. After boiling the potatoes for 20 minutes, then smashing them, drizzle with olive oil, then pan-roast them in a 400°F oven for 5 minutes.

Thanksgiving Rice with Lemon-Sesame Vinaigrette (page 48)

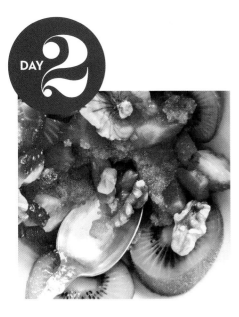

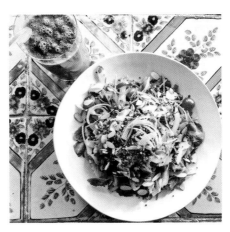

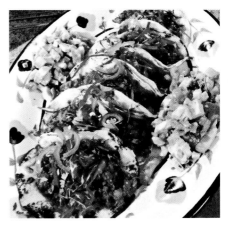

BREAKFAST

Amaranth with kiwi and strawberries (with a touch of maple syrup). I try variations on other days like changing the fruit and/or adding nuts and seeds. Amaranth is a naturally gluten-free "super grain" with a high complete protein content (it's actually a seed), containing calcium, magnesium, potassium, and iron. It lowers cholesterol, is a great source of fiber, and is the only grain with vitamin C! The Aztecs loved it, and so will you. Just follow the directions on the box and add your favorite fruit and/ or nuts. Drizzle with maple syrup if you want a touch of sweetness!

LUNCH

Baby Kale Salad with Balsamic Vinaigrette (page 41)

Green Smoothie (page 37)

DINNER

Vegetarian Tacos with Chipotle Sauce (page 47)

Quinoa Pico de Gallo Salad with Lemon-Garlic Vinaigrette (page 43)

Roasted Fennel (page 38)

Grilled Pineapple with Almond Milk Ice Cream and Maple Syrup Glaze (page 49)

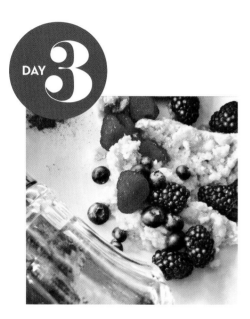

DAY 3

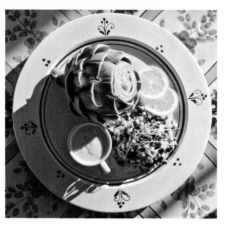

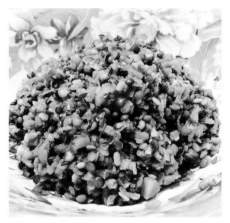

BREAKFAST

Ancient Harvest Quinoa Hot Cereal Flakes. It's gluten-free, non-GMO, and I like to call it the "Super Grain of Supermodels!"

LUNCH

Artichoke and mung bean salad. I like to cut the tops off my artichokes and steam them upside down till leaves are easy to tug off (not falling off!). Then add the leaves to some cooked mung beans and drizzle with olive oil.

DINNER

Lentil Curry Stew with Vegetables (page 46)

Roasted Cauliflower with Extra-Virgin Olive Oil and Curry Seasoning (page 45)

Brussels Sprout Fall Salad with Citrus-Almond Vinaigrette (page 40)

Coconut Pudding with Maple Sugar, Raspberry Sauce, and Dark Chocolate Chips (page 53)

DAY 21

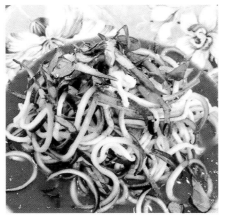

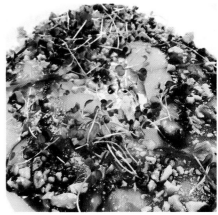

BREAKFAST

I often have dinner (leftovers) for breakfast. This morning, along with my coffee I had Brussels Sprout Fall Salad with Citrus-Almond Vinaigrette (page 40). It's one of my favorite salads that tastes extra great the next day, as the Brussels sprout leaves remain firm yet "marinated" in the oil and vinegar from the night before...yum! I added more fresh pomegranate seeds, which are packed with antioxidants and so many micronutrients. I also added slivered almonds, as they really stick with you throughout your morning so you won't experience blood sugar drops or midmorning fatigue.

LUNCH

Portobello, Roasted Peppers, & Microgreens Pizza (page 52)

"Zoodles" with Fresh Tomato Sauce (page 44)

Açai, Banana, and Berries Smoothie (page 37)

DINNER

Adzuki beans, cooked with shallots, garlic, and fresh herbs

Sautéed collard greens (Brazilian-style)

Barley salad with arugula, pomegranate seeds, red onions, and tomato (with champagne vinegar and Dijon mustard dressing)

Roasted golden beets, walnuts, and balsamic vinegar

Rhubarb and strawberry vegan cobbler

Satiating swaps: how to make any recipe healthier

Over the years, I've discovered that one of the easiest ways to make your recipes healthier is to replace not-so-good-for-you ingredients with ones that really add a lot of nutritional value. Sometimes the difference is undetectable, but sometimes I think it actually makes the dish taste even better than the original version.

Here are a few of Gabi's and my favorite ingredient swaps that you can use to boost the nutrition of any recipe.

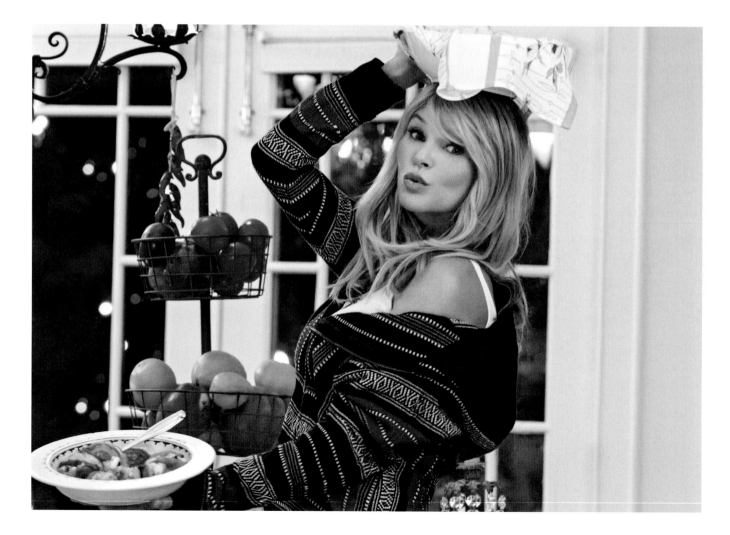

Unenlightened food	Enlightened food	
EGGS	**APPLESAUCE**	When baking, you can use applesauce to replace eggs (use ¼ cup per egg).
BUTTER	**COCONUT OIL**	Use it to replace butter in baked goods (and as a moisturizer on skin and hair!).
SUGAR	**MAPLE OR COCONUT SUGAR**	Gabi uses these instead of processed white sugar when making desserts. But remember that all sugars have the same chemical reaction within the body, so use less than the recipe calls for and add some nuts to slow the absorption of the sugar.
SUGAR	**DATES**	Pureed dates can be used to replace sugar altogether in baked goods.
MILK	**UNSWEETENED VANILLA ALMOND MILK**	Use it to replace milk in baked goods.
HEAVY CREAM	**CANNED COCONUT CREAM**	Use it instead of heavy cream for making whipped cream or chocolate sauce.
CHOCOLATE	**CACAO POWDER**	Mix it into recipes for chocolate icing or cakes to add beneficial antioxidants.

The enlightened way to lose weight

Even at those times when you want to drop a few pounds, there's still no need to embark on a crazy "deny-iting" plan. So many popular diet books advocate straying so far from your normal way of eating that it's unhealthy—not to mention unrealistic! If you're forced to give up too many foods, eat strange combinations, or subsist on nothing but juice, you'll undoubtedly gain weight back as soon as you return to eating normally. When my weight fluctuates—like after a holiday or during a stressful time—I simply adjust to eating smaller portion sizes of the healthy foods I usually eat, add more exercise, and stay focused on my goals. I CHOOSE to eat well because I know that I'll feel better during my upcoming photo shoot or special event. During those decades of being photographed in swimsuits, I learned a few things about how to get my body ready for the big reveal. So if you've got a week before heading off to a beach vacation (or a wedding, high school reunion, or other big event), following this modification of my normal eating plan (and sticking to these rules) will help you look and feel your best.

Drink plenty of water. Being even a little dehydrated can slow down your metabolism.

Cut out all white food—that includes sugar, flour, and things made with them.

(Yes, I mean bread, pasta, cookies, cake, etc.!)

Increase your fiber intake. Fiber not only digests slowly (so you feel fuller, longer), but it also burns more calories as you digest it.

Don't eat after 6 p.m., if possible.

Don't serve food family-style. Make up individual plates to keep portion sizes in check.

(And don't go looking for seconds!)

Eat more metabolism-boosting foods—such as citrus fruits, chile peppers, garlic, and green tea.

Eat an apple 20 minutes before a meal— it'll fill you up so that you feel satiated sooner.

Up your metabolism by doing some aerobic exercise for at least 20 minutes every day.

Do eat something small for dessert. It signals to your body that the meal is over, and makes you feel more satiated and not at all deprived. Opt for a small scoop of fresh fruit sorbet, a cup of grilled fruit, or fruit salad to satisfy your post-dinner sweet tooth.

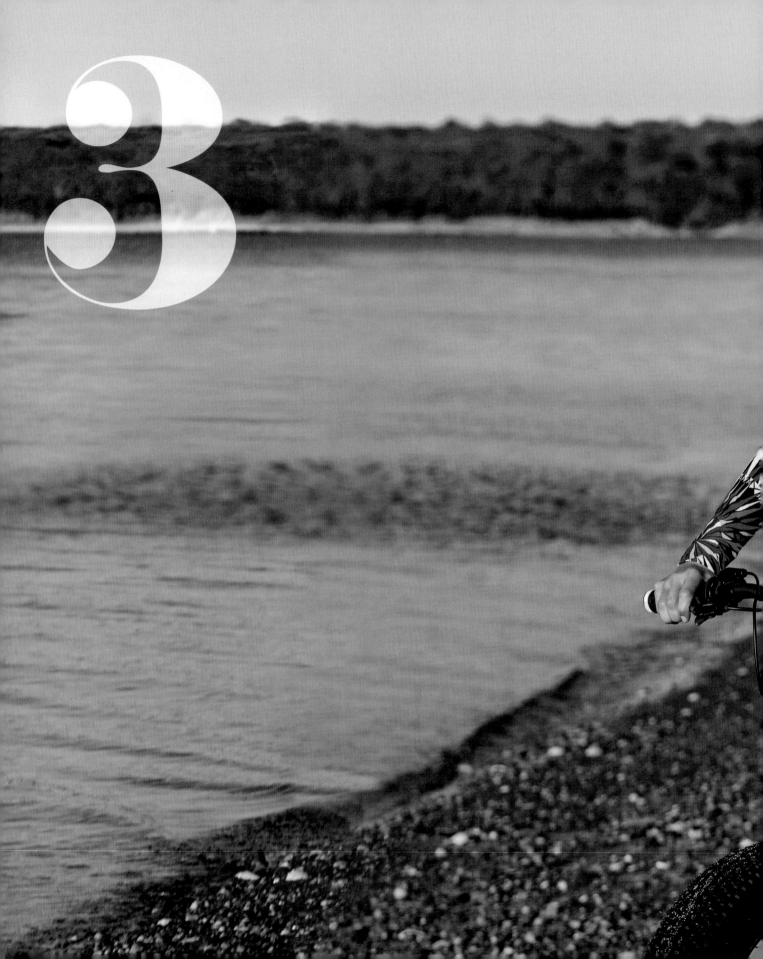

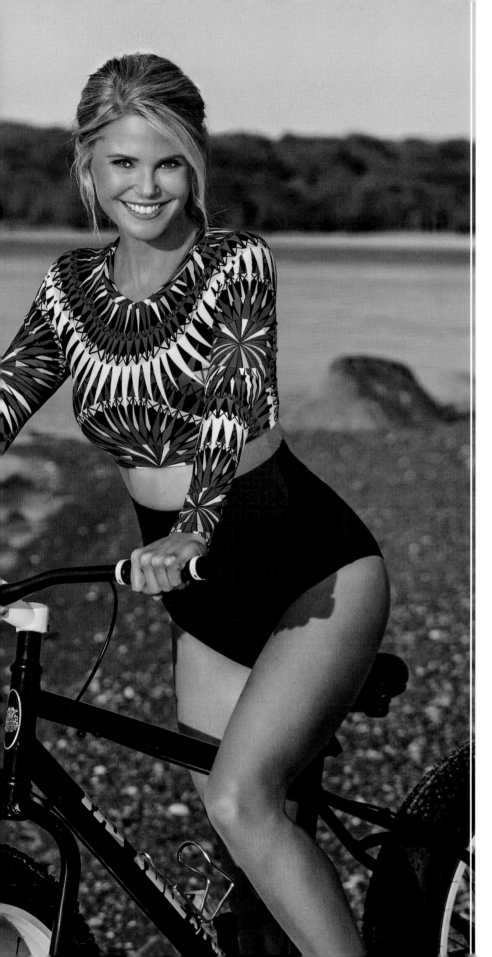

LIGHT UP YOUR LIFE WITH MOVEMENT

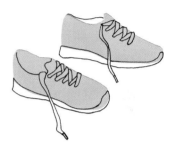

If you can't get motivated to exercise for your heart, do it for the ones you hold dearly in your heart.

Exercise has to be fun!

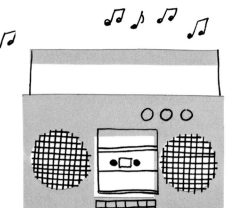

For me that means variety. I love to mix it up and do as many different activities as possible. That way I never get bored! The other crucial element is that you must get results. Results can take time, which is why finding ways to move that you enjoy every day is essential (that's what makes exercise fun, never a chore). And when you feel your jeans slip right on without a struggle, and you like the way the person smiling back at you from the mirror looks, that rewarding feeling will keep you committed to regular exercise.

Exercise will not only improve the way you look, your stamina, your endurance, and your overall health, but it also boosts your spirit. Exercise always puts me in a great mood. I know I am doing something good for myself, and that mood carries over into my day in so many positive ways. If I ever think about skipping my exercises, I just think about the great feeling of freedom, the joy of movement, the lightness and agility I feel after I do them and it motivates me to lace up my sneakers and get moving.

I cannot remember a time in my life when I haven't been active. I was lucky enough to grow up in California, right on the beach in Malibu. With the ocean as my backyard, I spent most of my days bodysurfing, paddling on my board, sailing, diving, surfing, running on the sand, or roaming the wild canyons and hills that looked down on the sea. Some of my best memories from my childhood are of bodysurfing with my mother—riding a wave in, running back out into the ocean and catching another one—for hours on end, listening to her infectious laugh. All the other moms would just sit on their beach towels in the sun, but not mine. And like mother, like daughter: I live by the ocean on Long Island where I raised my three children, and I'm still out there all summer long, riding waves with my kids.

I also love hiking because it combines my love of the outdoors with gorgeous scenery, and the rhythm of the hike becomes a kind of meditation that I find restorative. I enjoy skiing for the same reason. I feel so great at the end of a vigorous day on the slopes, and I know that I can eat everything on my dinner plate without any second thoughts or guilt!

Whether you're running, hiking, skiing, surfing, or even just going for a walk with friends, you are getting great exercise, but you'd never think you were because it's just so fun! And when you're having fun and doing different activities all the time, exercise never gets boring. Plus, doing different movements means you get the benefits of cross training, because you are constantly working different muscles.

It doesn't matter where you live— there are still ways to get outdoors and

QUICK TIP
THE POWER OF ECCENTRIC EXERCISE

There are two different types of strengthening moves—concentric and eccentric. Concentric is about shortening and contracting the muscles (think crunches), while eccentric is about strengthening while lengthening the muscles. "Eccentric contraction is our bodies' braking system," says my trainer, Ari Weller. "It is believed that most people could prevent slips and falls if they did eccentric training, because the muscles would know to turn on the brakes and stop the fall."

be active. I hope you can find a great trail in the woods, along a river, through a city park, near a bike path, or just on a pretty road. And since exercise is often more fun when you don't go it alone, explore options for finding workout partners—join a group that hikes together on weekends, or hook up with a friend who wants to try a new class at your local gym.

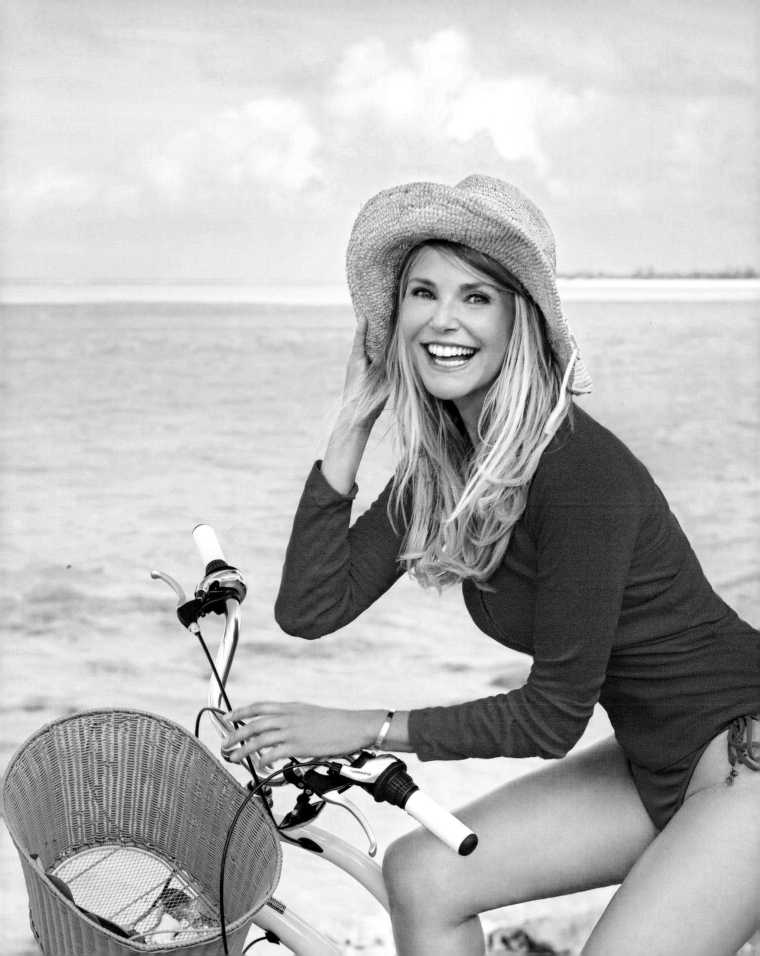

Injuries shouldn't stop you

What doesn't kill you might make you flabby—unless you get right back up again! My laundry list of injuries over the years is fairly impressive, but I've always been—and still am—determined not to let them get in the way of doing the things I love and staying in shape.
I've footnoted some of my major mishaps on my photo below!

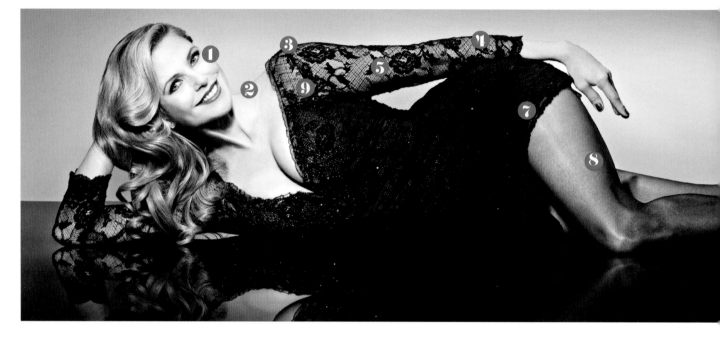

1. THE "BIRD" INCIDENT
Trying to save a wounded bird, I tripped, tore a muscle, and severely bruised the skin and bone near my left eyebrow.

2. THE BOATING ACCIDENT
I was sitting on the back of the motorboat when a rogue wave stopped the boat abruptly and I flew headfirst into the wall of the pilothouse, causing a compressed disk in my neck.

3. THE WEIGHT-LIFTING INJURY
Ruined my rotator cuff.

4. THE TUMBLEWEED TUMBLE
I fell off my spooked horse and landed smack-dab on my tailbone...broken!

5. THE SCHOOLYARD FALL
During a skipping race, I broke my arm in two places.

6. THE TRAMPOLINE INCIDENT
While doing flips, my leg went through the springs and I broke my foot.

7. THE CHAIRLIFT ACCIDENT
The sign said "Keep tips up." I didn't. My tips slipped under the snow and almost pulled my leg off, leaving me with a torn labrum.

8. THE HELLISH HELI-SKI CRASH
It was a brush with death that left behind scar tissue and bruising.

9. MY COMPETITIVE INSTINCT INJURY
Recently I aggravated an old shoulder injury while trying to keep up with my daughter Sailor at SoulCycle.

10. PAJAMA TRIPPING INCIDENT
Last year I broke my left foot by running full steam ahead and getting my big toe tangled in my pajama leg.

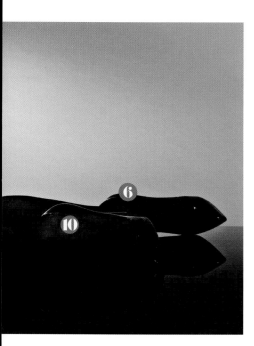

The list could go on...

But despite all these obstacles, when I got the once-in-a-lifetime offer to star as Roxie Hart in *Chicago the Musical* on Broadway at age fifty-eight, of course I said YES!!!!!

The secret to saying yes was to get moving, and to stay moving throughout the run. If I sit still for too long—at my computer, on a plane, at a restaurant, or in the car—I feel a little stiff and creaky on my injured right side when I get up. A perfect example of this would happen nightly during my run in *Chicago*. At the end of the show, Velma and Roxie have a long dance number, then are lowered down in a small elevator box and have to stay crouched there for several minutes till the final curtain falls. By the time I was able to uncurl myself, I would be so stiff I'd literally limp off to my dressing room!

Ultimately I had to leave the show as the pain from all my various injuries started to catch up with me. One of my mistakes during the run was not doing any other exercise—I thought the show was enough. And when I quit, I made the even bigger mistake of taking it easy and trying to rest up. Nothing could have been worse for me. The body will find ways to use other muscles in place of the one that hurts. Soon the aching muscle will get weaker as others take over. I got to the point where the pain was so bad in my right hip and left shoulder that I sought out second and third opinions. I had several doctors urging me to get hip replacement and rotator cuff surgery! I tried PRP (platelet-rich plasma) injections, which helped for a while, and hyaluronic acid shot into the joint, which was also effective but didn't last. Finally, and luckily, I found a much simpler, nonsurgical remedy that's really working for me—physical therapy.

The more I move, the better I feel. I just needed to know the right moves to get all my muscles working together again, and feeling improvement every day is pretty good motivation to keep moving! I work with two amazing physical therapists who've taught me the importance not only of continuing to exercise, but of learning how to do it correctly. This is not an area of your health where you should skimp—if you're injured, it's worth a few sessions with a physical therapist who can teach you how to continue to move through the pain without doing more damage, and how to heal and strengthen the injured areas. And even if you've never been injured (lucky you!), this information is vital for anyone who's looking to get or stay in shape.

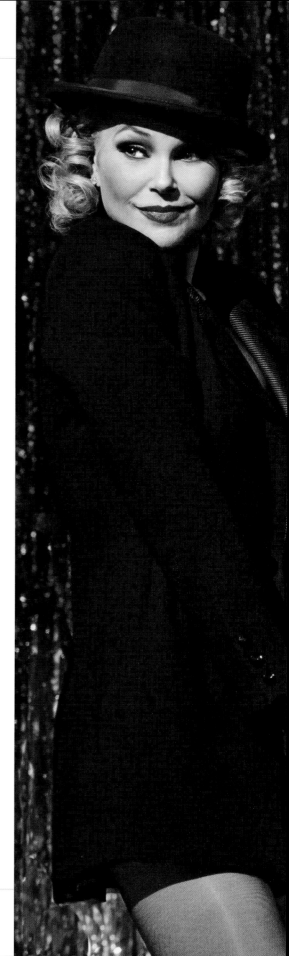

MEET THE MOVEMENT TRAINER:
Ari Weller

AND THE PHYSICAL THERAPIST:
Sinead Fitzgibbon

For the first time in my life I was actually starting to feel my age, because of all the aches and pains in my body from my active life. It suddenly felt like there were so many things I couldn't do physically, and then I went to see Sinead and Ari. They are literally turning back the clock for me by teaching me how to move and work through my injuries to repair my body and regain my strength. Doing my workouts with them (and taking the moves they've taught me home to do on my own) is making me feel stronger, fitter, and, most important, younger! So I've asked these miracle workers to share some of their wisdom with you too.

MASTER CLASS WITH ARI & SINEAD

"If you are dealing with injuries or physical limitations on movement, find a PT or trainer who can put you through a 'functional movement screen.' It's a simple series of movements that provides information to help target and strengthen weak areas in order to prevent injury." —SINEAD

"Results are in the details. You need to understand how the body works. Exercise isn't about quantity so much as it's about the quality of each movement." —ARI

"Crunches are about the worst thing you can do. They can cause injury to your back and your neck, and they are not actually very effective at strengthening your abs." —ARI

"Make sure your workout—and your everyday movements—covers a wide range of motions. You need to move in multiple planes in order to keep your muscles and joints lubricated and healthy. That's also why you need to mix it up. Doing something like a spin class is great exercise, but if you do only that, you're doing all your movement in a very limited range." —SINEAD

"The best thing you can do for your body is to keep moving. If we look at primitive cultures that don't sit as much as we do, they don't demonstrate the same incidence of arthritis and joint degeneration." —SINEAD

"Ninety percent of our lives is spent standing on two feet, so you need to learn functional postures that give you the strength to move safely." —ARI

"It's okay to 'feel your age,' but that shouldn't mean feeling old. Staying in shape isn't about feeling twenty when you're sixty, it's about being able to move without pain, be strong, and still be able to do the things you want to do." —SINEAD

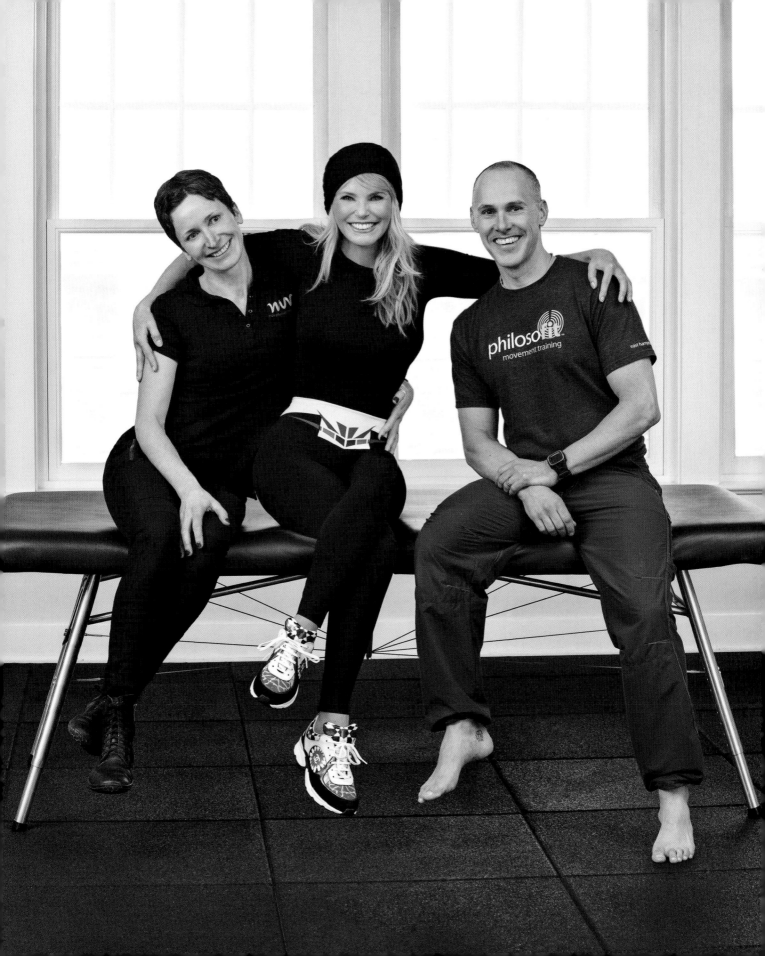

Ari's top 5 at-home moves

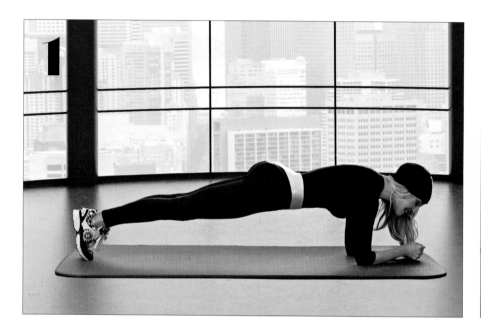

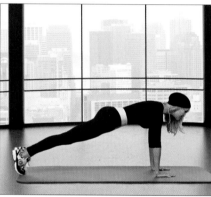

These five moves focus on building the eccentric strength needed to prevent injury and help you continue doing the activities you love.

DYNAMIC PLANK

TARGET: CORE

This plank is done on the forearms. Line the elbows directly underneath the shoulders (don't allow your shoulders to rise up toward your ears, and keep your abs braced to support your back). For more challenge, put your elbows 5 to 10 inches in front of your shoulders. This spreads the abdominal section out more, which calls for more abdominal engagement. Then try to "tug" (but not actually move) your elbows back toward your toes while engaging your quads and glutes. Hold for 30 to 60 seconds. The continuous dynamic tension makes this exercise much harder than a basic plank.

REVERSE PUSH-UP

TARGET: CHEST, SHOULDERS, ARMS

The setup is like a traditional push-up starting at the top. Keep the same dynamic tension as in the plank exercise (abs contracted, quads and glutes engaged), while slowly lowering yourself down to the floor as one solid connected body. While lowering (which should take 5 to 10 seconds), focus on continuously pressing your hands and feet into the floor—the slow lowering is what creates the eccentric contraction in the targeted body parts. Instead of pushing back up, just lower down to your knees and return to the push-up position. Repeat 8 to 12 times.

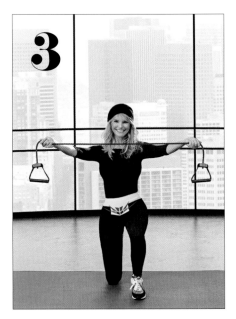

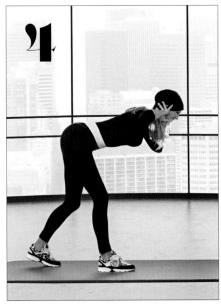

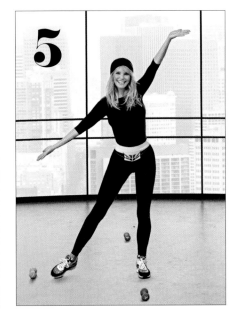

BAND PULLS

TARGET: UPPER BACK, POSTERIOR DELTOID

Hold a light- to medium-resistance band with both hands, approximately shoulder-width apart (narrower is harder), with palms facing up. Keeping your core tight, draw your shoulder blades toward the middle of your back, then start to stretch the band out with straight arms until the band is touching your upper chest. Slowly resist the band as it comes back to its starting position. Repeat 8 to 12 times.

GLUTE HINGE

TARGET: GLUTES, HAMSTRINGS

Stand in a split squat with one leg forward, one back. Bend the front leg at 20 degrees, keeping the foot flat on the floor. Bend your back leg at 20 degrees, with your heel up. Keep your arms crossed at your chest. Without changing the positioning of your legs, hinge your straight upper body up and over your front leg (without rounding your back). Think about trying to deepen the front hip joint as you hinge over. Take 3 to 5 seconds to lower down and 3 to 5 seconds to come back up. Repeat 8 to 12 times on each side.

QUAD CLOCK

TARGET: QUADS, HIPS

Imagine standing dead center in the middle of a clockface. Keep one leg stable and use your other leg to move around the clock. Start by simultaneously bending the stationary leg while reaching the moving leg out to barely touch an imaginary 12:00, then return to the start position. Do this 10 times in a row at 12:00, 3:00, and 6:00; when you get to 9:00, reach the right leg behind the bent/stationary left leg to touch 10 times. The bending of the stationary leg forces the quads and hips to eccentrically contract to stabilize the position. Repeat the sequence on the other side.

Swim the sand

(or trail, road, even treadmill!)

Even the classic jog needs a little spice once in a while, so here are some variations I've come up with to keep my workout interesting. I know these exercises sound silly (and look even sillier), but I promise the results are priceless. This simple concept came to me when I was getting ready to do the musical *Chicago*. I noticed that the second you add your arms (as a dancer does), you really up your heart rate. So, as I'm walking or jogging, I use my arms to do swimming strokes (like the crawl, breaststroke, and butterfly). Start by trying to do the crawl with your arms as you walk. Keep moving, checking your posture and standing tall. Are you getting out of breath? Great, it's working! I love this exercise because it improves your posture and is a great cardio workout. Try it with two-pound weights in each hand as another variation. Or you can move your arms as though you are a ballerina or an announcer proudly extending your arms to welcome the audience. In fact, imagine you *are* in front of an audience and focus on your posture—keep your shoulders back, stomach in, ribs down (feel it?). Now add big sweeping gestures with your arms. These exercises will help strengthen your triceps and prevent that flappy skin under your arms.

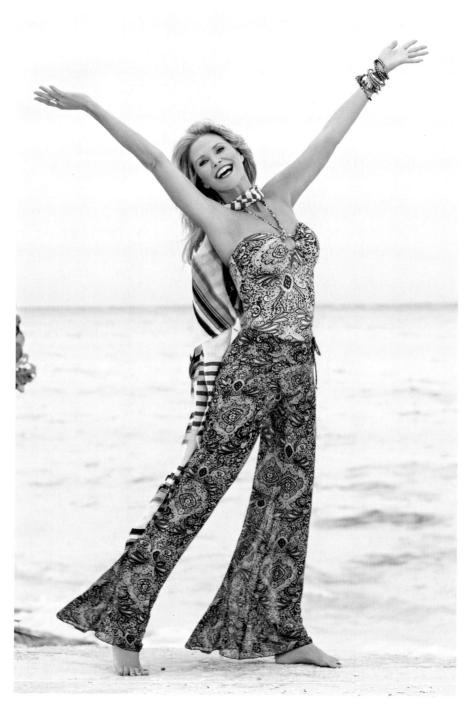

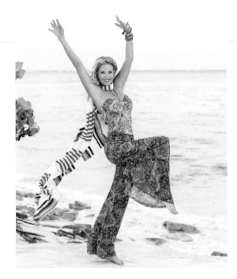

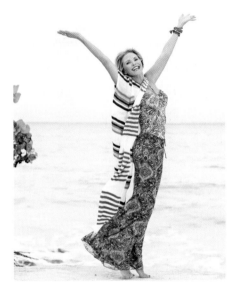

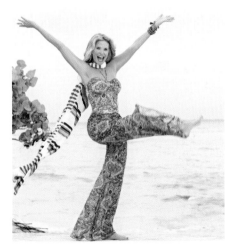

DON'T SIT STILL, EVEN AT THE OFFICE

If you need a reminder to keep moving, set an alarm every hour while you're sitting at your desk. When it goes off, get up and walk around the office, stand up to talk on the phone, or even slip outside for a stroll around the block.

QUICK TIP
TO STAY MOTIVATED, WRITE IT DOWN

I like to set smaller daily goals—I count as I do the exercises, and each day I like to add more so I am always getting stronger. It's almost like a game to write down how many push-ups I can do in a day or how long I can hold my plank pose. Then I try to do more the next day (and the next, and the next!). When a move gets too easy, challenge yourself to try a tougher variation.

QUICK TIP
RAINY DAY? TURN UP THE MUSIC AND DANCE!

Sometimes my daughter Sailor and I will blast music and try to do the latest dances. (Well, I TRY. She nails it and I provide the comic relief.) But we both end up drenched in sweat and laughing hard. And as we burn up "the dance floor," we are burning up calories too! You could also try a dance class—hip-hop, jazz, or something like Zumba—it's a really fun way to get your metabolism pumping.

ANTIAGING SECRET
KEEP MOVING! (DID YOU NOTICE THERE'S A THEME HERE?)

I like to say that I'm declining the decline! And I urge you to do the same. Even if you feel like you can't exercise or have gotten weak or out of shape, don't use that as an excuse to succumb to inactivity. If you're looking for a fountain of youth, exercise (and that can mean anything that keeps your body moving) is a good place to start.

PRODUCT RAVE

Ari and Sinead introduced me to the **Supernova massage ball**, and now I'm addicted to it. I use it before or after a workout (or while I'm at my desk or on the couch watching TV) to help release tight, overworked muscles—especially my hamstrings, calves, and lower back.

Yes, I really use it!
Total Gym— it works!

I've been a spokesperson for **Total Gym** since 1996, and yes, all you insomniacs, that's me (and Chuck Norris) on TV in the middle of the night! Even after eighteen years, it is still my go-to workout. I love that I can work my whole body without leaving the house. Depending on my mood and what my body feels like, I can use the Total Gym to do an intense strength training workout, some gentle stretches, or even Pilates exercises similar to what you'd do on a reformer in a studio. And it's always lengthening and strengthening your muscles at the same time, both preventing injury and keeping muscles strong.

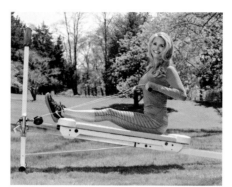

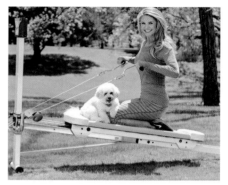

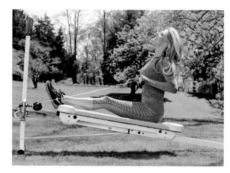

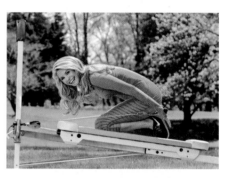

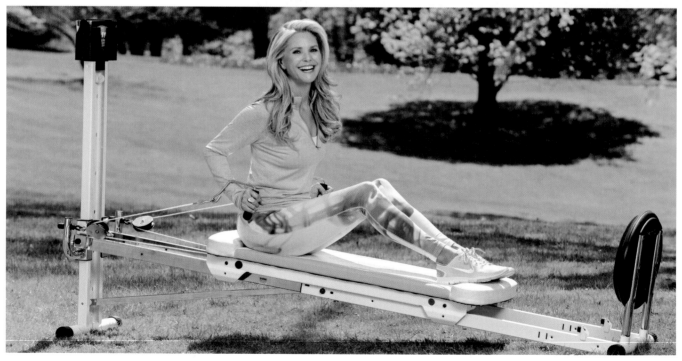

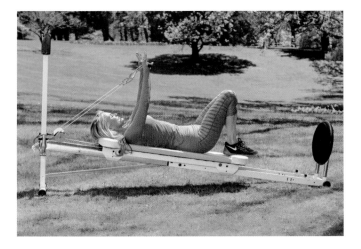 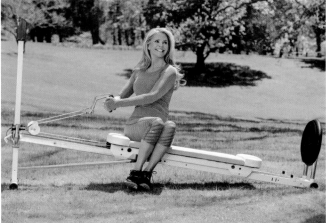

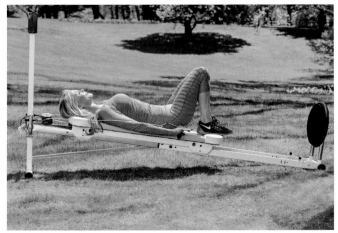 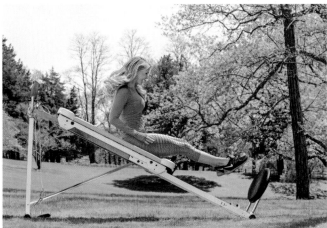

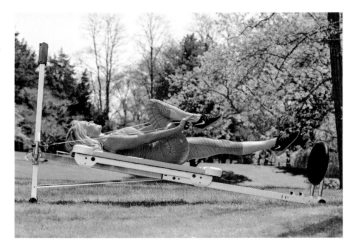 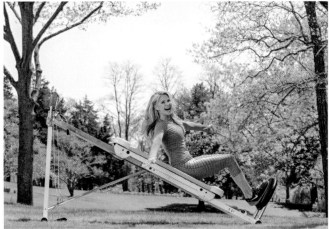

Time to multi-taskercise!

On those really busy days when you can't find time for even a quick workout, there are a few sneaky ways to multitask and fit in some exercise along with your morning routine. When my life gets too packed to go to a class or for a run on the beach, or even to use my Total Gym, I "multi-taskercise." I try to capitalize on those times when I'm a captive audience—like when I'm blow-drying my hair, brushing my teeth, washing and chopping vegetables, watching TV with the kids—and incorporate as many quick exercise moves into that time as I can.

QUICK TIP
THE HIGH-HEEL WORKOUT

To keep my leg muscles in shape to walk in heels when I need to, I do this simple "multi-taskercise" when I'm brushing my teeth, drying my hair, or putting on makeup. Alternate balancing on one foot and then the other to strengthen those tiny, stabilizing muscles in your feet and ankles. As you progress, try going up onto the ball of your foot and balancing to work the calf muscles as well.

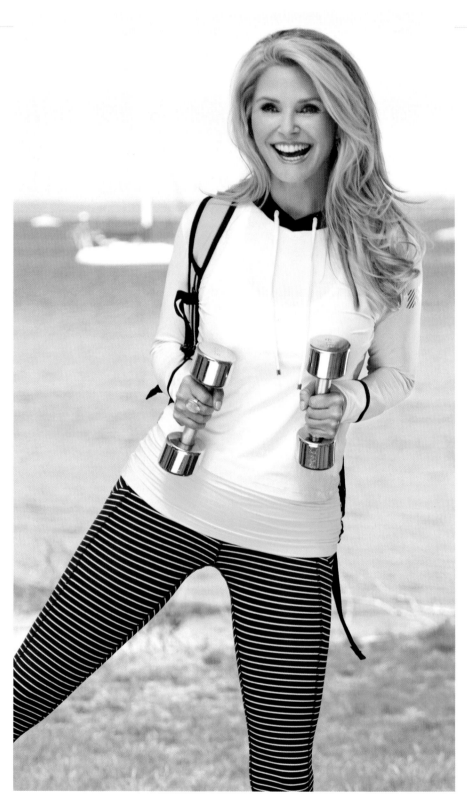

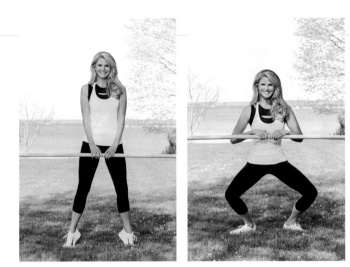

PLIÉS

It's easy to fit in a couple of sets of 10 pliés while drying my hair (my hair takes a long time to dry!).

LUNGES

Here's another move I do while drying my hair. Make sure your knee never gets in front of your foot, and follow through the full range of motion that's comfortable for you.

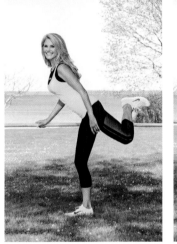
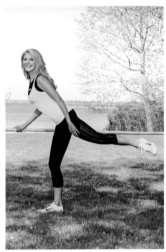
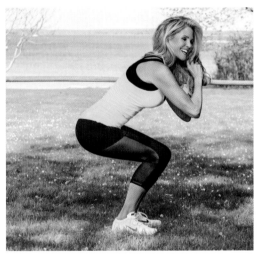

STANDING LEG LIFTS

When I'm brushing my teeth, I bend one leg behind me and press up with my heel for a set of lifts (be sure to do the same number on both sides). Or I'll lift my leg straight up in front of me, making sure to tighten my abs and squeeze my butt while I hold it there for a few seconds. And any time you're doing something on one leg, it's great for improving your balance too.

CHAIR SIT

While I'm drying my hair, I'll pretend I'm sitting in a chair, even though there's no chair there. It's a great way to strengthen and tone the thighs and butt.

A workout for your brain

Exercise is physical, for sure, and there are many obvious benefits for our bodies. Working out keeps our muscles strong and toned, helps us manage weight by keeping our metabolisms high so we don't have to count calories, and keeps our heart and lungs healthy. But don't underestimate what exercise can do for your brain too. Research over the years on the benefits of exercise has found that it can improve your memory (and even decrease your risk of Alzheimer's), help you sleep better, lower your stress levels, and improve your mood. I know that within seconds of starting a workout, my mind feels clearer and my body feels more relaxed—especially if I'm lucky enough to exercise outside. It makes me happy just to be outdoors! And when I'm walking, hiking, or running, it almost feels like meditation. My mind becomes so peaceful and calm. Whatever worries I had before heading out suddenly seem less important. It really puts everything into perspective. And afterward, thanks to the endorphins released during a workout, I get a boost to my mood that can last all day!

When I do yoga, I always take a few minutes at the end of my practice to calm myself and try to quiet the inner voice that's stressing out about my to-do list and everything else. I find that even just taking five minutes for myself can have a huge impact on how I manage my stress. Regular meditation can help lower the levels of the stress hormone cortisol, which your body produces. Excess cortisol is bad for you in many ways, not the least of which is that it can lead to fat being stored in your belly. I've seen this connection firsthand! During a particularly stressful period in my life, when I wasn't making time for myself, I noticed myself gaining weight in my stomach for the first time.

So find five minutes away from your phone, away from the kids, away from your desk. Sit quietly, focus on your breathing, and just "be" with yourself. Your mind and your body will thank you for it.

QUICK TIP
BOOST YOUR METABOLISM

The amino acid L-carnitine has been shown to help improve the way your body metabolizes fat. Try to add a little of this supplement to your diet to make your workout results even better.

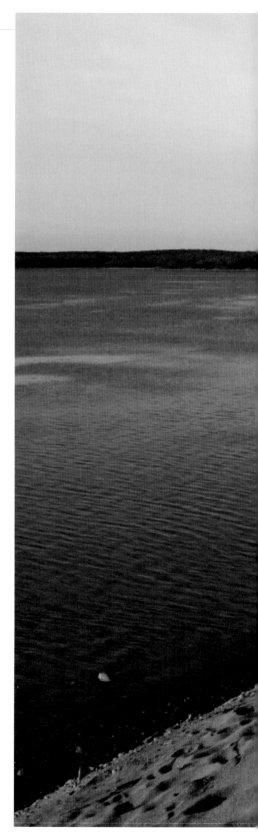

**Have a nice Namaste!
And don't forget
to move that body!**

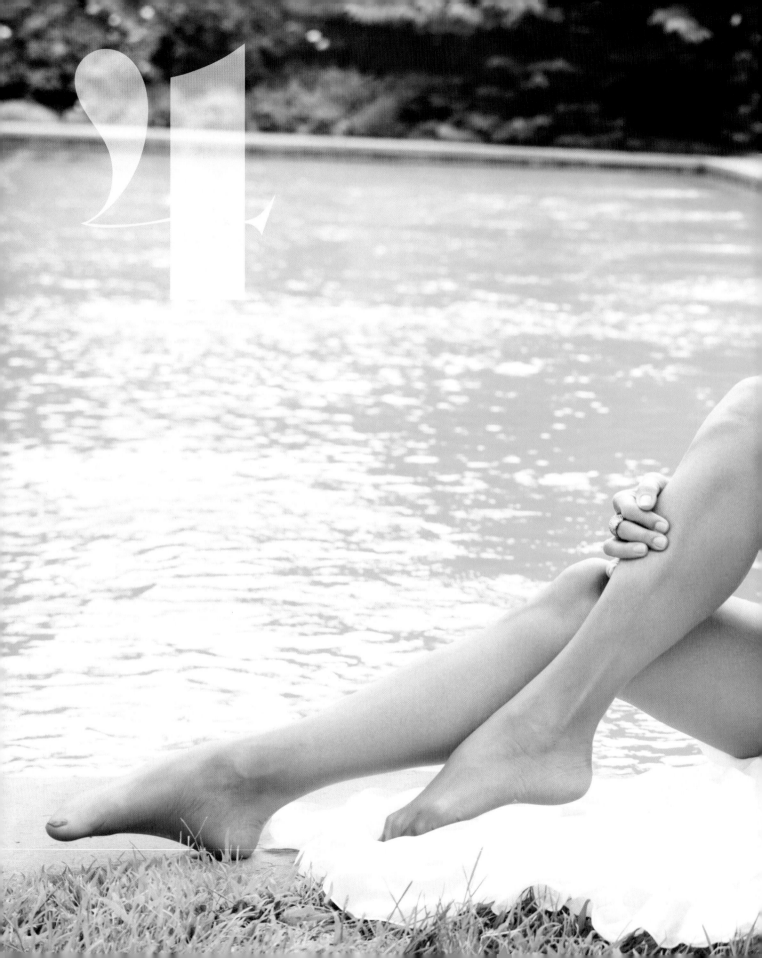

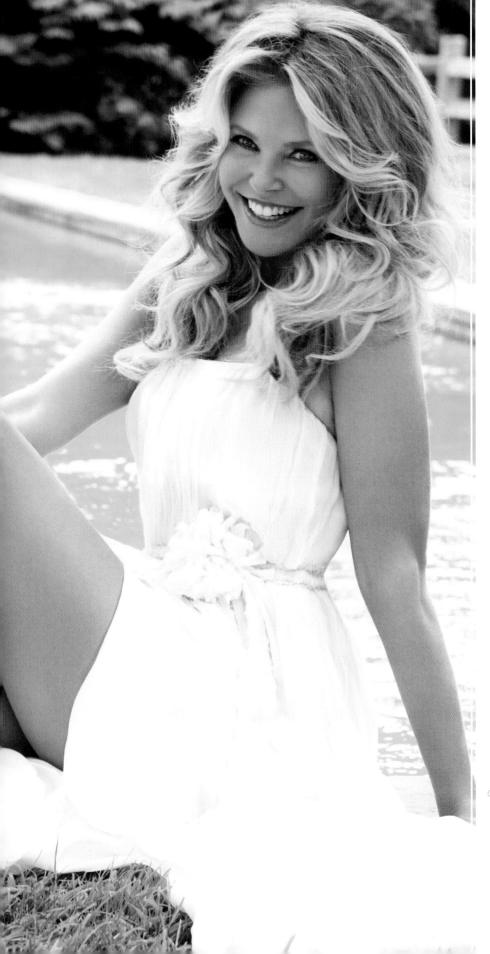

LOVE THE SKIN YOU'RE IN

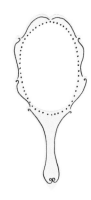

Curvy women are real women. Skinny women are real women.

What makes us "real" people is not the shape of our flesh but our basic humanity.

–Hugo Schwyzer

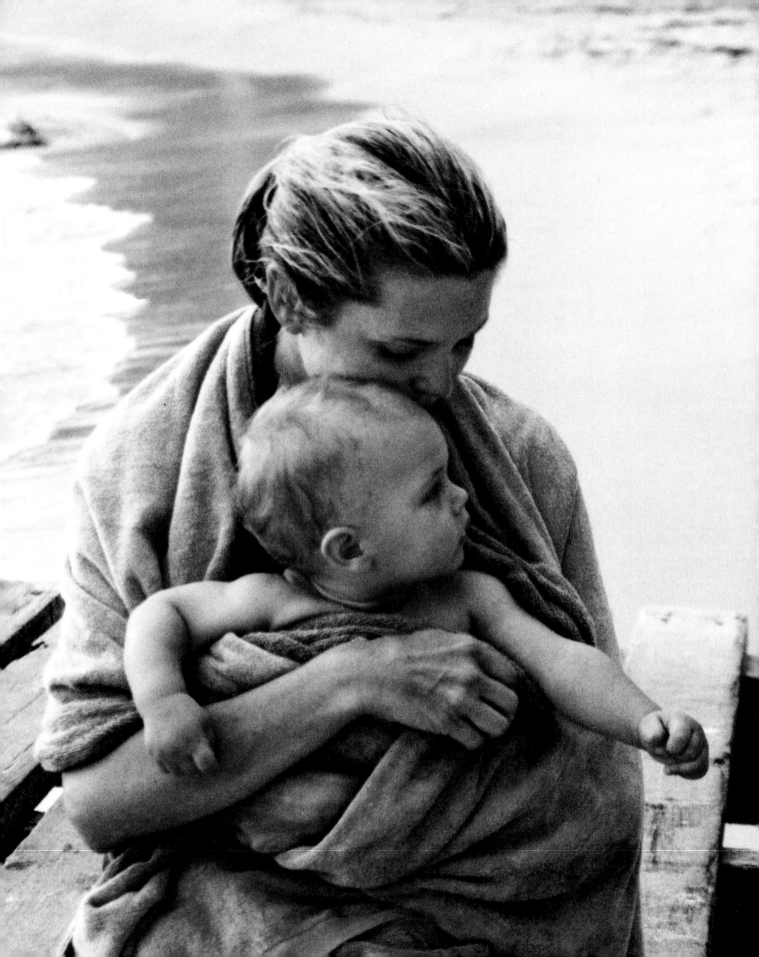

TRULY BEAUTIFUL SKIN

radiates with the glow of good health—no matter your age! And that starts with a healthy diet. Eating well is a fabulous way to help your skin every day—with every bite. That's why when people ask me my big secret to looking younger than my age, I reply, "Eating right will keep it tight!"

Seriously, though, good skin is a combination of good nutrition, a great 24/7 skin care regimen, skilled dermatologists, and a few makeup tricks (more on those in the next chapter). This simple formula is guaranteed to make you feel great about putting your best face forward—so let's get glowing! I know, those are some corny puns, but if you found it "punny," that's great, because maybe it made you smile—which is one of my favorite beauty tips! You really can't underestimate the power of a smile. Smiling gives an instant lift to your mood as well as your face. So smile as you finish this chapter, or move through your day, and feel how it lightens your mood and how others pick up on your infectious smile. Joy is contagious and very, very attractive. In fact, a smile is the best thing you can put on your face to always look your most beautiful.

My sonshine, Jack

ANTIAGING SECRET
Foods to avoid

SUGAR is one food to avoid if you're worried about the health and beauty of your skin. We are learning more and more about just how much havoc it wreaks on the skin. The latest buzzword is something called "glycation"—a process that starts as sugar is broken down in the body, and is destructive to the collagen and elastin in your skin, causing premature aging.

PROCESSED WHITE FLOUR is high on the glycemic index—and foods in that category have been linked to acne breakouts.

SALT causes tissues to swell and look puffy (hello, undereye bags!).

ALCOHOL can be dehydrating, which is never a good thing for skin. So drink in moderation and always balance out a glass of wine with a big glass of water.

FEED YOUR FACE
The top foods for great skin

Every day scientists are giving us more good news about how proactive we can be in influencing our health and appearance just by eating the right foods. I gobble up articles about nutrition. I not only find them fascinating, but the more I know about how food is powering and protecting me, the more inspired I am to make healthy choices. It's nice to feel so powerful just doing something we all love...EATING!

Some foods in particular pack more of a punch when it comes to boosting your natural beauty. Turn the page to see which superfoods are especially good for your skin, and be sure to add plenty of them to your daily diet.

Superfoods for your skin

WALNUTS

These nuts are a great source of omega-3 fatty acids, which help strengthen the skin and also attract and hold moisture so that skin looks plump, healthy, and well hydrated. I always keep a little plastic bag with walnuts in my purse to nibble on throughout the day.

PAPAYA, STRAWBERRIES, & KIWIS

These fruits are all rich sources of vitamin C. Vitamin C is one of the most important vitamins for your skin—it helps promote collagen growth and prevents free radical damage.

BERRIES

Fruits and vegetables in deep, rich hues (like blueberries and blackberries) are potent sources of free radical–fighting antioxidants.

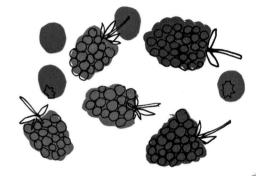

CARROTS

Carotenoids have been shown to help fight aging by protecting skin from UV damage, and carrots are one of the best sources of this nutrient.

RADISHES

This root vegetable contains vitamin C, sulfur, and silicon—all of which support collagen production and help keep skin supple and elastic.

GREEN TEA

This beverage is naturally full of antioxidants that help fight the cellular damage that contributes to wrinkles and skin aging.

RED BELL PEPPERS

Raw in a salad or roasted in the oven, red peppers are one of my favorite ways to get vitamin C. Yum! One medium pepper contains more than 200 percent of your daily vitamin C requirement.

TOMATOES

Tomatoes are full of lycopene, which is an antioxidant and is also anti-inflammatory. The best way to get it is to cook the tomatoes, so it's a wonderful excuse to eat pasta and tomato sauce—just watch out for the salt, which can make you puffy and contribute to wrinkles under your eyes. (But I must say that laughing and eating pasta are two of the most fun ways to get wrinkles, and I'll very happily take them!) Pink grapefruit is another good source of lycopene.

SWEET POTATO

Vitamin A is essential for skin health and helps prevent skin aging by promoting collagen repair and growth, and sweet potatoes contain high levels of it. I like to quarter a sweet potato and roast it. I keep plenty stocked in my fridge as a healthy snack that satiates my sweet tooth too.

WILD SALMON

For those who eat fish, salmon has a lot of benefits, like selenium to help protect you from the sun and lots of omega-3 fatty acids to keep your skin soft and moisturized.

OYSTERS

These shellfish have zinc to renew and repair your skin, and they are delicious with champagne! (Nothing like a fun night out with friends and laughter to keep you young!) And if you have left-over champagne, pour it on your hair to make it shiny.

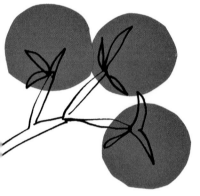

BIOSIL SUPPLEMENTS

I'm a firm believer that you should get as many of your nutrients as possible from your food, but a good supplement can also work wonders. I started taking **BioSil**, and I'm amazed at the difference I've seen in my nails, skin, and hair. The nutrients in it help the body build more collagen, the substance that keeps skin firm, plump, and smooth.

There are also nutritional boosters to put into shakes and salads, like wheat germ, brewer's yeast, chia seeds, flax-seeds, oats, and powders like **Activz**. These foods give your body and your skin a boost of extra nutrients!

BRAZIL NUTS

They are high in selenium, a mineral that helps repair skin cell damage and prevent premature aging.

TOFU, SOY MILK, & EDAMAME

The magic ingredient in these tasty treats is isoflavones, which may help stop the breakdown of collagen.

SPINACH

This leafy green has lutein and other carotenoids, which protect you from sun damage. Note: Make sure to store your spinach in the light until you eat it to help it retain vitamins like C, K, and E.

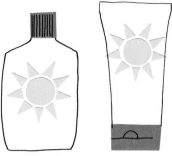

The good-skin essentials

How you care for your skin at home is really more important than you can imagine. Just remember, you're in charge of what's on your skin twenty-four hours a day. This is your chance to treat your skin with ingredients that will replenish and nourish it. Your daily regimen should include cleansing, protecting, treating, and repairing.

SUNSCREEN

I know you've heard this before, but the absolute, number one, single most important thing you can do for your skin is to wear sunscreen. Every single day, rain or shine! Did you know that even on overcast days, 80 percent of UV rays can still penetrate the clouds and reach your skin to do damage? Plus, there are infrared rays—which come from anything that emits heat, like the sun, ovens, hair dryers, computers, cell phones, and radiators—that are also harmful to your skin. What happens when any of this radiation hits the skin is that it penetrates deep below the surface where it generates free radicals that attack your collagen and alter skin cells. That means skin ages faster (sagging, wrinkling, and getting sun spots), and the alterations in the cells can also lead to skin cancer. The Skin Cancer Foundation recommends using a daily sunscreen that provides broad-spectrum protection and has an SPF of at least 15 (for spending longer periods outdoors, they suggest SPF 30 or higher).

I am well aware of the damage the sun can cause. I grew up on the beach in Malibu, and I was out in the sun in my bikini every day. As a child, I was always brown as a berry! And when I grew up and got a job as a model, getting a tan was part of the job description. I would show up at some exotic beach location for a swimsuit shoot, and be told to spend the first day getting tan. I used to joke, "Can you believe how lucky I am to be getting paid to work on my tan?" In my first beauty book (published in 1983), I actually provided lots of "helpful" tips on how to get a great tan. Yikes! I am so sorry!

Not surprisingly, all those years on the beach have left their mark. I can see the demarcation line on my thigh where my sarong ended—the part the sarong covered still looks fairly smooth, but the exposed areas are a bit blotchy. But luckily it's never too late to repair, restore, and protect skin from further damage. (And don't forget to see your dermatologist at least once a year to check for skin cancer.)

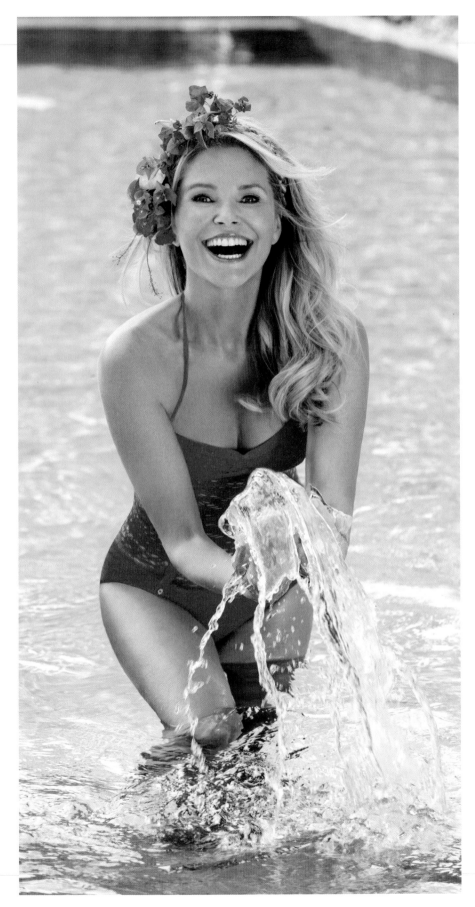

EXFOLIANTS

Exfoliation is another very important part of my daily skin care routine. I started scrubbing when I was just a teen and I never let up. I remember reading that the reason men age so well is because they shave every day, and that daily scraping of their skin leads to faster cell turnover and more vibrant skin. So I have always been a big exfoliator. I absolutely LOVE the smooth feeling of my skin after a scrub! Back in the day, I used some pretty rugged scrubs—they were kind of like rubbing gravel on your face. I still exfoliate every single day, but now I opt for a gentler touch. I like to apply my scrub to dry skin, rub it in, then rinse. (If you have sensitive skin, add water before you scrub.) Your skin will feel refreshed and oh so smooth—ready to really receive the moisturizer. Exfoliating also makes your foundation and blush go on more smoothly because there are no dry or rough spots for it to grab on to.

RETINOLS OR PEPTIDES

The other key to making the most of your skin care routine is using products that help restore skin according to your body's own biorhythms. Nighttime is when the skin does its best repair work. By applying restorative products like tetrapeptides with antiaging ingredients that act at the cellular level as you sleep, your skin can work on rebuilding collagen while you rest. So never go to sleep with your makeup on, or you'll miss out on an opportunity to get so much done while you're sleeping!

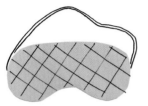

TIPS TO BANISH A BREAKOUT...FAST!

I rarely break out, but if I suspect a pimple might pop up, I rush to treat it. If I am quick enough, I find I can stop it from happening. I put a tiny drop of cortisone cream over the spot and apply a dab of drying facemask on top to seal it in. Or I'll use the **Proactiv** wash, but only on the problem spot, then a touch of the toner, and then a dot of the mask just exactly on the spot and leave it there for anywhere from 15 minutes to an hour or even overnight. This method stops a pimple in its tracks, but for it to work you MUST be quick. As soon as you feel it, RUN! (But if you break out regularly, don't use my cortisone trick because frequent use can thin the skin—and these days we all need a thick skin! LOL!) A dab of toothpaste will also help get the red out of a pimple. And don't underestimate the power of clay to draw out impurities and help dry up a pimple fast. My favorite is bentonite clay.

DON'T EAT IT, SCRUB WITH IT

What to do with all that sugar you're no longer eating because it's bad for your skin? Make a face or body scrub! For the body, just add sugar to 1 tablespoon coconut oil till the mixture turns into a scrub consistency. For an antiaging facial scrub, add it to green tea.

GET YOUR ZZZS

I really NEED my beauty sleep! My skin is the first thing to betray my lack of sleep. I believe that a good night's sleep is mandatory if you want to really feel and look great. Ways to help make that happen: Keep your bedroom cool and dark. Make sure there is no light from TVs, computers, tablets, or cell phones—the blue light they emit interferes with sleep patterns. (If you must read your phone or tablet in bed, wear a pair of blue light–blocking glasses.) Wear a sleep mask if you can't get the room dark enough. Use a humidifier to keep the air moist and a white noise machine to block out sounds. It's worth all that effort to create a peaceful place so you can dream sweet dreams and awaken refreshed and ready to SHINE!

KNOW WHAT'S IN YOUR PRODUCTS

If you're worried about what you're putting on your skin, I recommend going to the **Environmental Working Group**'s website, ewg.org. They have a cosmetic database called **Skin Deep**, listing every product imaginable and rating the ingredients based on their safety.

PRODUCT RAVE

Elizabeth Arden Eight Hour Cream is a must for any dry situations—hands, cuticles, feet, lips, face. I used to smear it on my face for every airplane ride. It's a classic!

PRODUCT RAVE

I hope to add a waterproof version of my sunscreen to my skin care line soon, but for now I'm still testing ingredients and formulations. So when I'm spending time in the water, I reach for **Neutrogena Wet Skin Sunscreen Spray, Broad Spectrum SPF 85+** (and a hat!).

My skin care secret

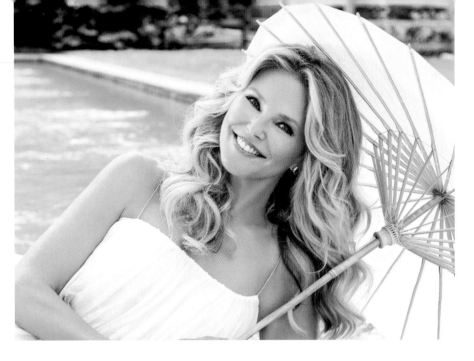

I'll always be an outdoors enthusiast, so I need the broadest sunscreen protection possible, and my sunscreen also needs to be the perfect base for the makeup that my modeling jobs require. It's got to be effective, yet pure and gentle. Plus, I need it to be antiaging, tightening, repairing, moisturizing, and smoothing, and I wanted all that in ecofriendly packaging too. A tall order, I know! And when I couldn't find it, I decided to create it—along with a complete collection of other products for cleansing, protecting, replenishing, and restoring skin. I pulled together top experts to help me produce the exceptional skin care products I wanted. I reached out to dermatologist Dr. Doris Day and cosmetic scientist Dr. Mindy Goldstein—both renowned leaders in their fields—and I asked them to come up with what I believe to be the ultimate product line, **Christie Brinkley Authentic Skincare.** The day creams contain proprietary ingredients that provide the most comprehensive sun protection available—protecting skin not only from UVA and UVB rays, but also from infrared radiation, which represents 54 percent of the radiation reaching earth. And antiaging ingredients, such as a bio-copper complex, are truly effective for helping to fade sun spots, firm skin, and reduce the appearance of wrinkles—providing results on par with retinol, but without the irritation and sun sensitivity that retinol can sometimes cause.

I wanted every layer of my skin care to stay on message, and by that I mean that I wanted each product to fortify the next and work together. My skin care line is 100 percent vegan and cruelty-free, and all the products are formulated without parabens, formaldehyde donors, mineral oil, alcohol, propylene glycol, and nano-sized particles. Everything is as organic and natural as it can be without sacrificing elegance and efficacy.

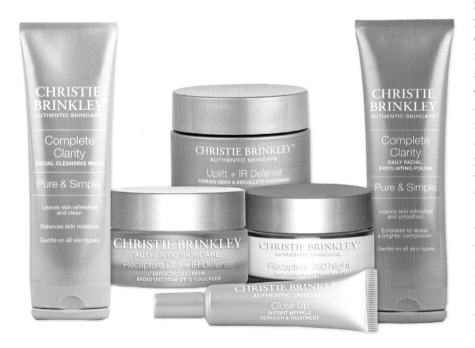

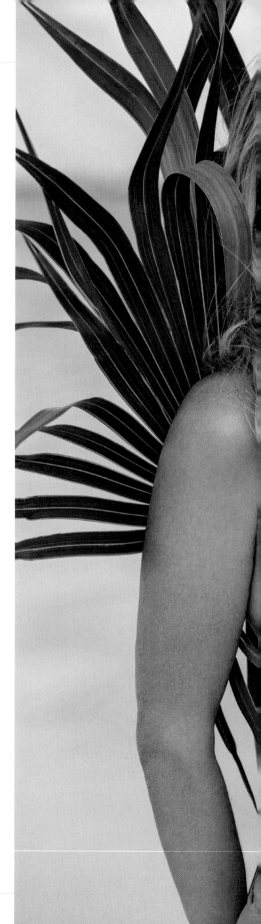

Don't bake, fake

So now we all know that tanning is about the worst thing you can do for your skin. It will make you look older sooner and increase your risk of getting potentially deadly skin cancer. But luckily there are some great products out there that fake a tan quite naturally! I don't like going to spray-tanning salons because I don't like the idea of breathing those particles, so I self-tan at home. If I am going to the beach and I want to have a sunny, beachy look, I opt for tinted moisturizer and bronzer for my face, and I love some of the newer body moisturizers that produce a subtle "tan" with daily use. They are so gradual they never streak, making them as easy to use as moisturizer! I always buy both formulas—I'll start with the "fair to medium," then start mixing that with "medium to dark," and finally progress to all "medium to dark." Doing it this way is foolproof. I also always exfoliate prior to using any tanners so they don't deposit too much color into dry skin spots. And for my back, I just use a spray tanner.

Here are a few of my favorites:

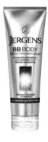

Jergens BB Body Perfecting Skin Cream (This great product moisturizes, evens out skin tone, and even helps firm skin!)

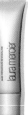

NARS Pure Radiant Tinted Moisturizer Broad Spectrum SPF 30

Laura Mercier Tinted Moisturizer, Broad Spectrum SPF 20 for face

Skin-sational ideas

I always moisturize not just my face but also my neck, ears, décolletage, and the backs of my hands. (Wish I had started doing that part sooner!)

For my body, I alternate creams that subtly tan (see page 90 for self-tanner brands I like) with ones that firm (like **Clarins Extra-Firming Body Cream**).

Apple cider vinegar can restore your skin's pH after a sunburn. And aloe vera gel will help take away some of the heat and sting (so do cucumbers and cool tea bags).

Use lavender essential oil as a hand sanitizer. It's natural, gentle, and smells great too!

Soak black tea bags in hot water, remove excess water, and cool them in the fridge for about twenty minutes, and then place them over your eyes for five minutes or so to reduce puffiness. And yes, it's true...hemorrhoid cream will help shrink up and tighten the skin under the eyes too.

Staying hydrated is so important for your skin, so not only do I drink lots of water, I also eat foods that pack a lot of moisture—like cucumbers, melons, and other fruits. Herbal or green tea is another great way to stay hydrated, plus get some extra antioxidants.

Speaking of water, did you know if you moisturize with **Evian Mineral Water Spray** or other spritzers (like I always do on an airplane), you need to blot the water after you spray it on your face? If you let it air-dry, it will actually dehydrate your skin because the evaporating water will pull additional moisture from your skin.

Don't smoke! Not only is it bad for your health, it's horrible for your skin. You'll get smoker's lines around your mouth that will make you look old before your time.

I keep arnica gel in the fridge to soothe bumps and bruises. It stops the pain and helps bruises heal faster. And the sublingual arnica tablets really help speed recovery!

If you have a cut and you're worried about scarring, try the new silicone gel bandages. The way the technology helps heal without leaving a mark is amazing!

Does she or doesn't she?*

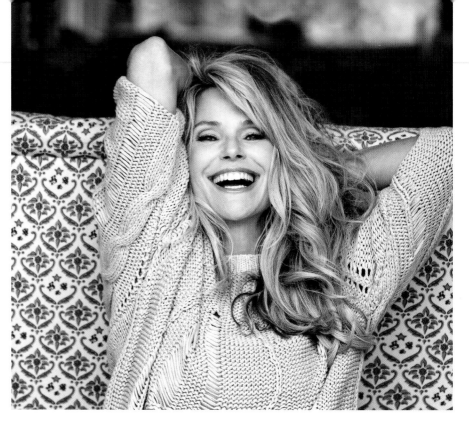

Only her dermatologist knows for sure!

It's an exciting time in dermatology. It seems that nearly every day there's another innovative cosmetic treatment promising to erase years off the skin. Some procedures may even help stave off skin cancer in the future while beautifying you today. And a study published in November 2014 by the American Medical Association found noninvasive and minimally invasive procedures like fillers, neurotoxins, lasers, and other energy devices to be generally safe. The researchers concluded that these procedures are "safe when performed by experienced board-certified dermatologists," and that "adverse events occur in less than one percent of patients and most of these are minor and transient." Well, that's great news! But I couldn't agree more that the safety and efficacy of these treatments depend entirely on the doctor you choose. So regardless of how upbeat that study's conclusions may sound, this is still an area of beauty that should be approached with caution and thoroughly researched. (You'll find some important information about how to choose a qualified doctor later in this chapter.)

I remember that when I was a kid there was a stigma attached to women who dyed their hair. Today, thankfully, we have so many more beauty choices—and much less judgment attached to them! So I say, if something bothers you, it's okay to tweak it. Don't like your gray hair? Cover it up (or even make it pink or purple if you choose). And the same goes for skin wrinkles, sagging, and discoloration. With today's menu of cosmetic treatment options, you can pretty much pick and choose which things bother you and do something about them.

We could have a whole discussion here about the external pressure we all face to look a certain way. But nobody can tell you what's right or wrong for you, and hopefully you are not looking at cosmetic treatments as a way to become something or someone you are not. The best results aren't a total transformation, but nearly imperceptible tweaks that make you look like you—just perhaps a slightly younger version of you! This is an area where less really is more.

Being in the beauty industry, I hear about everything that's available and I see lots of great results. I am always interested in what might benefit my skin. And now, at sixty, I've dabbled in several different treatments—with varying degrees of success.

My one brush with having Botox injected into my forehead was a disaster. Looking back, I don't even know why I bothered. My forehead looked fine—until I got the Botox! Instead of making me look serene and relaxed, it took the arch out of my eyebrows and made me look sad. I actually started to feel depressed too! My face lacked expression, and I couldn't wait for the Botox to wear off. I never tried it again, at least not in my forehead. But more recently I noticed vertical bands in my neck that were particularly obvious with side lighting.

I didn't like them, so I inquired about what could be done, and apparently, the easiest way to address this issue was to inject a small amount of Botox into the "strings" in my neck. It worked wonders to relax those muscles, and it also tightened my double chin area and jawline. The good thing about using Botox in this area is that you don't have to worry about any expression being lost or changed—you just get the improvement.

I've also tried a laser treatment that was nothing short of miraculous. Last summer I got poison ivy and was left with noticeable discoloration on my face. After just a few treatments with a Clear + Brilliant laser (which wasn't painful and didn't make my skin more red or flaky), the discoloration was mostly gone and my skin tone was back to normal. The process also stimulates your body to produce collagen, so I got the added bonus over time of my face looking fuller and more youthful.

Skin-tightening devices, like the

TriPollar Apollo, which uses radio frequency waves, can do amazing things without any surgical lifting. It sounded too good to be true, and when I had it done, it felt like a hot stone massage. I was interested in the toning effect, which was imperceptible to the point of wondering if what I did notice was a placebo effect. But the faint horizontal lines above my knees were indeed gone after the treatment. This is something I would try again!

I have used fillers in super-tiny doses—and just like makeup, the best ones are imperceptible. I've used them on an indentation on my forehead from a playground accident, and on marionette lines around my mouth. But you must use a very small amount because over-filling removes your contours and gives you a flat face! If you have a pockmark, a wrinkle that you feel distracts, or a scowl that does not reflect your attitude, filler can be a good solution.

My panel of experts

There are so many different ways now to give your face or body a fresh look—from a variety of fillers to replace the volume, to lasers, radio waves, light waves, and even treatments that use growth hormones from your own blood to generate new cells. But I am not a doctor and I don't claim to be any sort of expert in this area, so the last thing I would want to do is recommend that you try (or avoid) any particular treatment. Those decisions should be between you and your dermatologist. What I can do is share some information about what treatments are currently available to help you educate yourself and be better able to make the right choices for your skin. So let's go to the experts to fill you in... (Pun intended! Ha!)

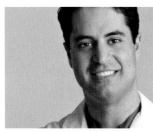

DR. ROBERT ANOLIK
Practices at Laser & Skin Surgery Center of New York. Clinical assistant professor of dermatology at NYU School of Medicine and Weill Cornell Medical College.

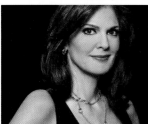

DR. DORIS DAY
Practices in New York City at Day Dermatology & Aesthetics. Clinical associate professor of dermatology at the NYU Langone Medical Center.

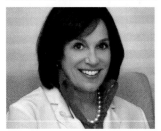

DR. ELLEN GENDLER
Practices in New York City. Clinical associate professor of dermatology at NYU Langone Medical Center.

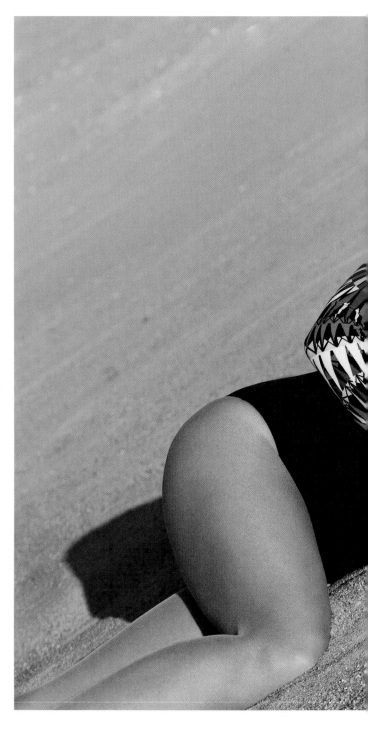

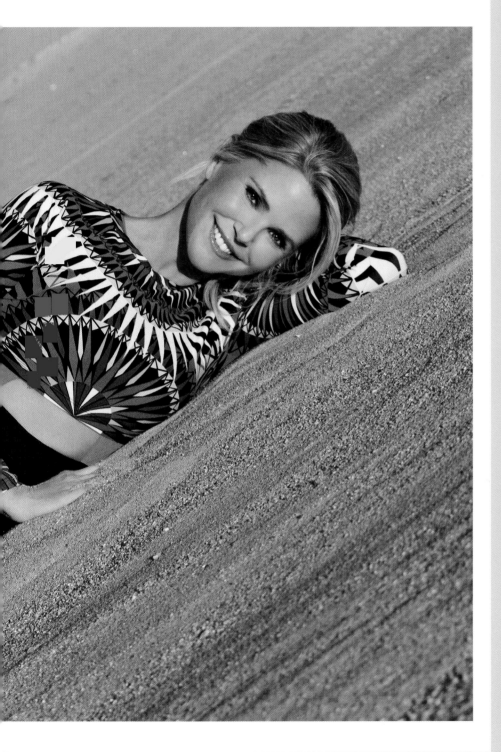

DR. FREDRIC BRANDT: A TRUE SKIN GENIUS

When Dr. Brandt passed away in 2015, the beauty industry lost a real antiaging innovator and I lost a person whose opinion and expertise I trusted. He was an artist who looked at each face individually, listened to each personal story, and offered his talent and words of wisdom to make each lucky patient feel beautiful from the heart up. In his hands, Botox and fillers, used in minute doses, were tools that erased years—while leaving his patients looking naturally refreshed. He was a visionary, always working to find ways to finesse treatments to make them even more effective, while also researching and experimenting to find the newest, next best thing. One of the last times I saw him, I asked what was on the horizon that he was excited about. He described a new process he was investigating that he was convinced would revolutionize antiaging. It's a treatment that involves drawing a patient's blood and isolating the growth factors and anti-inflammatory factors. Those are then injected back into the skin to stimulate your own collagen, smooth skin, and improve overall texture...almost like aging backward!

In addition to his incredible skills, Dr. Brandt was a kind and wonderful man who entered every room singing Broadway tunes and standards. The last time I saw him he was singing one of my favorites, "Smile." He said it was one of his favorites too. Appropriate for a man who lived to help women look in the mirror and smile.

What do each of you consider the go-to, most-bang-for-the-buck treatment for someone who wants to look refreshed, rejuvenated, and like a very natural, younger-looking version of themselves?

DR. DAY: "I love using filler to restore lost volume to the face. It's not just about chasing lines and filling in holes. When you truly understand facial anatomy—and what's going on in the face that's causing those wrinkles—you can put filler in just the right places and lift the entire face."

DR. ANOLIK: "The technology for laser rejuvenation has come so far that you can now achieve tremendous results with minimal downtime. The treatments exfoliate the skin surface to help brighten the complexion, erase sun spots, and can even potentially eliminate precancerous skin changes. Lasers have the ability to amplify the quality and quantity of collagen in the skin, which helps tighten pores, smooth out skin texture, and address fine lines and wrinkles."

DR. GENDLER: "I would say that the combination of injectable fillers with Botox gives the biggest bang for your buck. The treatment doesn't take long, the results are almost immediate, and you'll see many months of improvement. The filler helps correct the natural volume loss that occurs with age, while the Botox addresses the fine lines in the forehead, around the eyes, and can give a lift to the brows. The two treatments together can give the face back a very youthful look."

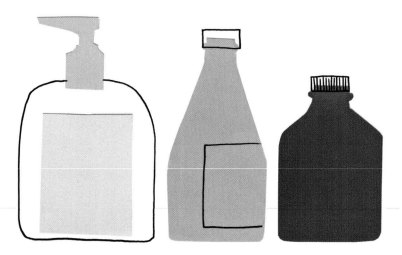

What new things are coming out that you're especially excited about?

DR. DAY: "There are more skin-tightening devices in the works that will more effectively treat submental fullness in the neck (also known as turkey neck!) without a surgical neck lift. They can tighten loose skin and stimulate new collagen production that reduces sagging. Hopefully they will give better, more consistent results than those currently available (like Thermage and Ultherapy). And a new injectable treatment for submental fullness, called Kybella, is now available that literally breaks up and eliminates the fat under the chin."

DR. ANOLIK: "The new lasers being developed just keep getting more effective. I've recently started using the PicoSure laser, and it's a game-changer. It delivers a more rapid pulse of energy to the skin to provide results that are faster and more effective. It does an amazing job of breaking down pigment— making it ideal for removal of tattoos and sun spots. But we're also seeing amazing results for antiaging. After one treatment, we're seeing textural changes to the skin comparable to more invasive rejuvenation lasers that require five days of redness, peeling, and downtime after treatment."

DR. GENDLER: "Younger women are beginning to accept that keeping their skin looking beautiful and remaining healthy is a maintenance process, more than a corrective one, so I think the trend will be toward quicker, smaller procedures that can easily be done on a regular basis. There are new fillers that will be better at addressing lines around the lips and restoring a youthful appearance to the mouth. New lasers that give long-lasting effects without unreasonable downtime. And new topical treatments that use retinoids to rejuvenate the skin in less irritating formulas."

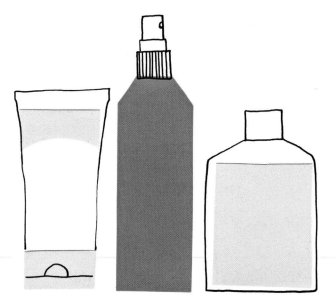

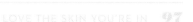

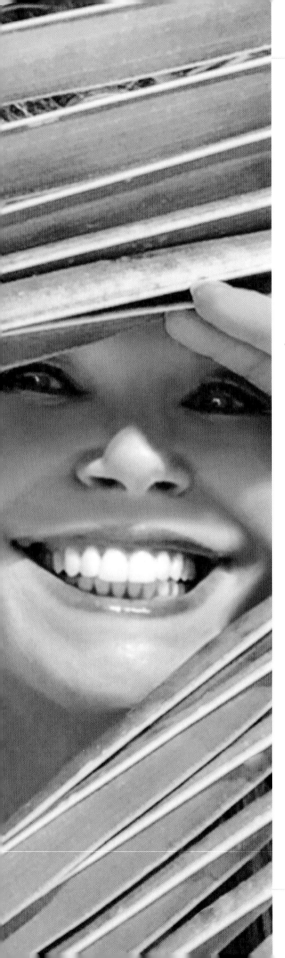

The most common antiaging and skin-rejuvenating procedures

FILLERS

Brand names such as Voluma, Juvéderm, Restylane, Sculptra Aesthetic, and Radiesse

Dermal fillers are used (as the name implies) to fill in places that have lost volume due to aging. That means they are effective not only for filling up wrinkles and indented scars, but can also restore volume to the cheeks, hands, and other areas that have lost their youthful fullness. Results are immediate and can last for six to twelve months. The way fillers are used has been changing—with results that are much more natural looking. Cutting-edge dermatologists no longer just fill up wrinkles. Instead, they have learned how and where to inject to actually restore the volume of a youthful face. This can give the overall face a lift and diminish fine lines while helping to re-create the face of your younger self.

NEUROMODULATORS

Brand names such as Botox, Xeomin, and Dysport

These are used to relax the excessive muscle contractions that can lead to crow's-feet, forehead furrows, and rope-like bands in the neck and jawline. In the right hands, Botox (and similar products) can produce a lift to the brows and forehead. But beware of doctors who overuse or misplace it—that can cause brows to droop (which happened to me!) or lift too much, which creates a surprised look. Results start to become visible within forty-eight hours and the effects can last for three to six months.

WILL IT HURT?

When it comes to cosmetic treatments, there's some truth to the old adage "No pain, no gain." Injections, lasers, and energy treatments are rarely completely pain-free. But the good news is that any pain involved is usually minimal, rarely lasts much longer than the treatment itself, and can be easily mitigated. Talk to your doctor if you are planning to get a treatment, because he or she can recommend some pain-relieving steps to take before you arrive for your appointment. Topical lidocaine gel can be applied to any area that's about to be treated to help numb the skin (great for injections, lasers, and energy treatments). Normally, you'll want to apply it about an hour before treatment. If you're worried about more pain, ask your doctor if taking a drug like Valium or Vicodin is an option (and be sure to arrange to have someone drive you to and from the appointment if you do take it).

QUICK TIP
KEEP BRUISING AT BAY

To minimize bruising from injectables, you need to stop taking any medications or supplements that thin your blood. Cut out aspirin two weeks prior to your appointment, and starting two to three days prior, skip any NSAIDs (like ibuprofen), fish oil, vitamin E, ginkgo biloba, and alcohol.

LASERS

Brand names such as Fraxel, Clear + Brilliant, and PicoSure

Lasers deliver energy to the skin in a variety of ways and to achieve a variety of results. There are lasers that specifically target broken blood vessels or help break up pigments to remove tattoos and birthmarks. There are ones that work to erase brown spots (and even precancerous lesions) caused by sun damage and ones that go deep into the skin to stimulate collagen to get rid of fine lines and enhance skin texture. For most conditions, you can expect to do a series of monthly treatments to achieve optimal results, then follow up with one to four treatments a year for maintenance.

SKIN-TIGHTENING TREATMENTS

Brand names such as Thermage, Ultherapy, and TriPollar Apollo

These devices deliver energy (in the form of radio frequency or ultrasound) deep into the skin to heat it and stimulate the production of new collagen. As new collagen forms, skin gets firmer and less saggy. Different devices can be used on the face, neck, décolletage, stomach, knees, and so on. Results develop over a period of two to six months after a treatment, and can last for a year or more.

FAT-REDUCTION TREATMENTS

Brand names such as CoolSculpting

These devices can't deliver quite the same results as surgical liposuction, but they can provide significant reduction in fat (on the abdomen, thighs, back, etc.) noninvasively and with no real downtime. They work by cooling the fat cells underneath the skin, which triggers a permanent elimination of those cells. Results are typically seen four to six months posttreatment, and, provided you maintain your weight and fitness, the results can be long lasting. A new device called Cellfina was recently approved for treating cellulite—it works by making micro-incisions under the skin to cut the bands that hold the dimpled fat together. So far, data has shown that results can last a year or more.

Finding a qualified dermatologist

I'm fortunate enough to have access to some of New York City's top dermatologists—the ones you see quoted all the time in women's magazines. So I know that when I put my face in their hands, I can trust that the treatments they suggest are right for me, and that they have the skills needed to administer them safely and effectively. But what should you do if you don't live near a major city and don't have access to the top doctors?

Once again, I asked my panel of experts for their advice, and here's what they had to say:

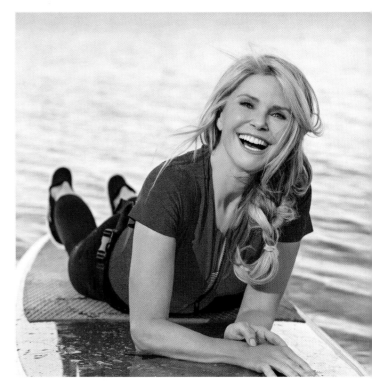

CHECK CREDENTIALS

Just because someone has "MD" after their name doesn't necessarily make them the right person to go to when you're seeking a cosmetic procedure. You need to see a doctor who is board-certified by the American Board of Medical Specialties (ABMS) in dermatology or plastic surgery—specialties that include years of study in the anatomy of the skin, lasers, and surgery-related cosmetic improvement. The ABMS oversees physician specialists in twenty-four medical specialties, including dermatology and plastic surgery, and is viewed as the gold standard of certification. You can check the ABMS website certificationmatters.org to see if your doctor is listed. Be wary of other organizations that allow doctors and others to purchase a so-called "board certification," potentially after attending just a one-day seminar or taking an online course.

DO YOUR HOMEWORK

If you read or hear about a procedure that sounds like something you'd like to try, do a little research on it. Find out what you can from reliable resources about how much the treatment should cost, what kind of results you can expect, how long they last, and whether or not it's recommended for your skin type and condition. Then, if the doctor you see tries to tell you something contradictory, you'll recognize it as a potential red flag.

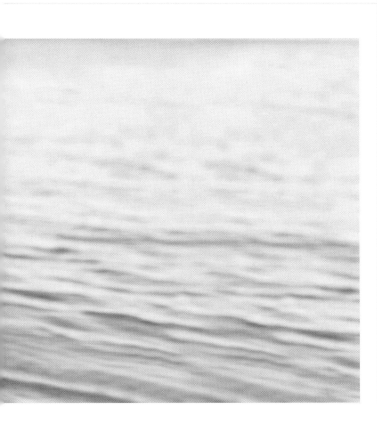

STAY IN THE KNOW

New antiaging ingredients, treatments, and procedures are being developed all the time, and I can only guarantee that what we've told you in this chapter was the latest word up to the publication of the book. So if you're considering a treatment—or hear about a new one that piques your curiosity—ask your dermatologist about it or check out these websites for up-to-date information:

American Society for Dermatologic Surgery
www.asds.net

American Academy of Dermatology
www.aad.org

Real Self
www.realself.com

ASK QUESTIONS

Don't be afraid to speak up. Ask about a doctor's credentials and their experience with specific procedures. And find out who will actually be administering the treatment. Is it the doctor or a less experienced aesthetician or nurse practitioner? Also, be sure you and the doctor are on the same page and share the same vision of the improvements you hope to achieve.

DON'T PRICE SHOP

It can be tempting to look for a deal, but save your bargain hunting for something other than cosmetic procedures. Shopping based on price alone could lead you to an inexperienced practitioner or to a procedure that's not right for your skin. And while most cosmetic procedures are very safe in the right hands, in the wrong ones, they can still have dire consequences. Disfiguring burns from lasers, fillers that cause painful infections, and hyperpigmentation caused by inappropriate use of lasers or other skin resurfacing techniques are not uncommon. And someone offering cut-rate Botox or fillers may be using diluted (or potentially even counterfeit) product. One risk of diluted Botox is that it can more easily travel to other places after injection—leading to drooping eyebrows or eyelids, for example.

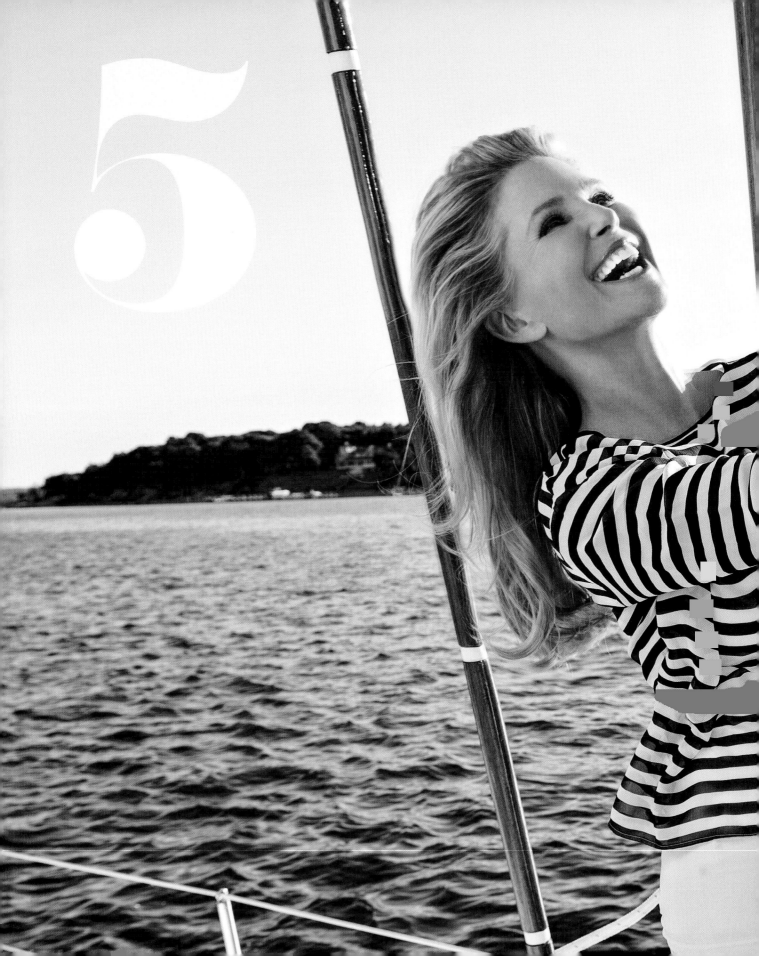

5

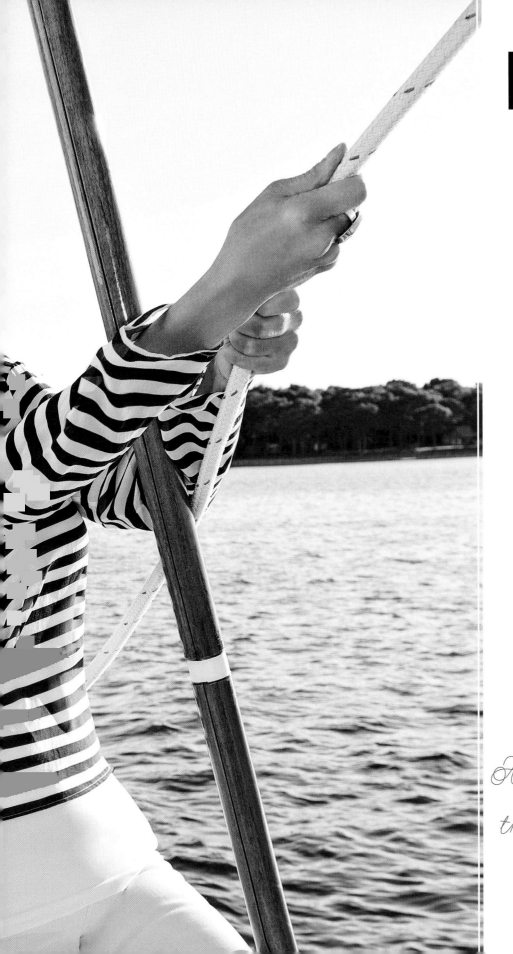

MAKEUP
MAGIC

A smile & sunblock are the two best things you can put on your face.

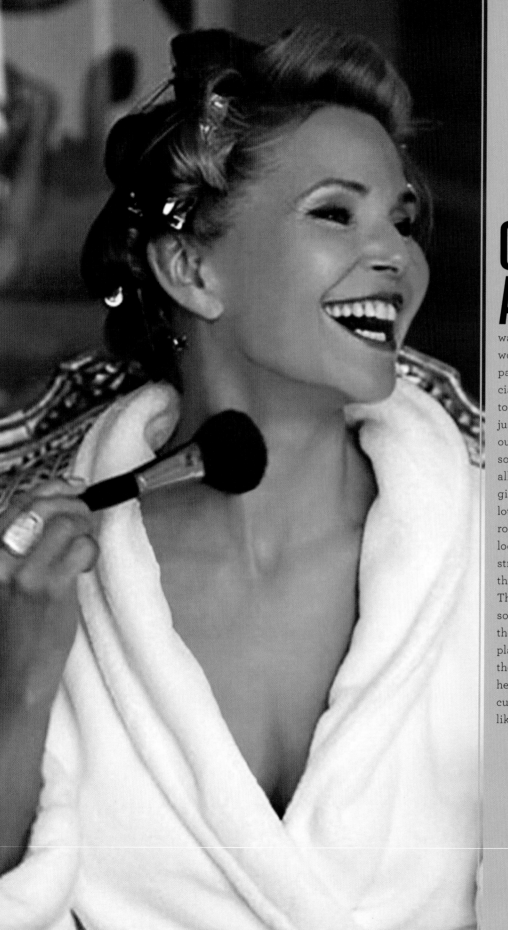

ONCE UPON A TIME,

way back in the day, when I took my first wobbly high-heeled steps as a model, part of the job description for commercial work like catalogs was that we had to do our own hair and makeup. And not just one look for the day. Oh no! Each outfit required a different look—sporty, sophisticated, demure, you name it! So all the girls would dig through their giant bags looking for their favorite lotions, potions, powders, pins, and rollers to create all kinds of different looks. It was fun, but it could also be stressful—especially to try to pull it off in the limited time we had between shots. Through trial and error I learned a lot— sometimes the hard way. For example, the first time I used an eyelash curler, I placed my unsuspecting lashes between the clamps and squeezed hard until I heard a popping noise! There on the curler were all my lashes, looking just like a set of falsies!

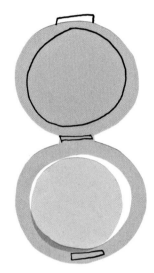

But with help from the professional models around me, the editors on the shoots, and trying to copy the way professional makeup artists painted my face in Paris before I moved back to the United States, I learned how to take my "blank canvas" face and make it into the required "daytime," "evening," "sophisticated," "natural," and "sporty" looks. And over time, I figured out what made me look good on camera (warm, pink blush and taupe and brown eye shadow) and what didn't (blue eye shadow, white undereye concealer). I even learned tricks for keeping makeup in place while modeling the warmest winter clothes during the heat and humidity of a sweltering August day in NYC's Central Park (think about snow and icicles, and use lots of blotting papers!), and how to define my features yet look like I had no makeup on, while splashing in the surf in a bikini.

Later, as more and more professional makeup artists came on the scene, being a model no longer meant carrying that heavy bag of magic tricks. I could sit back and let someone else work on

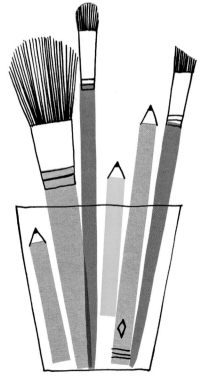

my face for a change. But I definitely didn't sit idly. I saw each opportunity to be in the hands of a professional makeup artist as a chance to learn as much as I could about new products, application techniques, and tricks of the trade. Over the years, I have placed my face in the hands of some of the biggest names in the business, and I want to share some of the tips I've learned (and am still learning) from these talented experts. I don't know why people always call these sorts of tips beauty "secrets," when it's the stuff everyone loves to talk about and share with each other. We all want to know how to make our eyes look bigger, our skin more flawless, and how to get lipstick to stay on through dinner! And who better to talk makeup with than a few of my favorite professional makeup artist friends? So read on to find out all the juicy details that will transform your routine and give you the skills you need to create model-worthy makeup every day!

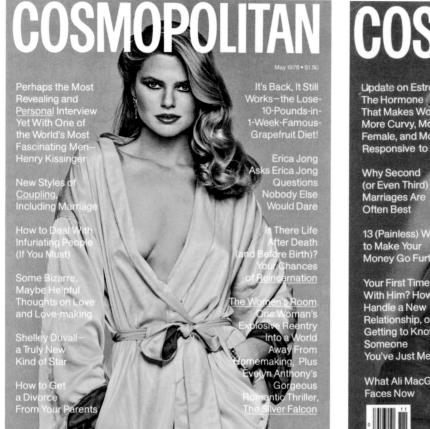

COSMOPOLITAN

May 1978 • $1.50

Perhaps the Most
Revealing and
Personal Interview
Yet With One of
the World's Most
Fascinating Men—
Henry Kissinger

New Styles of
Coupling,
Including Marriage

How to Deal With
Infuriating People
(If You Must)

Some Bizarre,
Maybe Helpful
Thoughts on Love
and Love-making

Shelley Duvall—
a Truly New
Kind of Star

How to Get
a Divorce
From Your Parents

It's Back, It Still
Works—the Lose-
10-Pounds-in-
1-Week-Famous-
Grapefruit Diet!

Erica Jong
Asks Erica Jong
Questions
Nobody Else
Would Dare

Is There Life
After Death
(and Before Birth)?
Your Chances
of Reincarnation

The Women's Room.
One Woman's
Explosive Reentry
Into a World
Away From
Homemaking, Plus
Evelyn Anthony's
Gorgeous
Romantic Thriller,
The Silver Falcon

Makeup by Way Bandy

COSMOPOLITAN

November 1979 • $1.50

Update on Estrogen:
The Hormone
That Makes Women
More Curvy, More
Female, and More
Responsive to Men

Why Second
(or Even Third)
Marriages Are
Often Best

13 (Painless) Ways
to Make Your
Money Go Further

Your First Time
With Him? How to
Handle a New
Relationship, or
Getting to Know
Someone
You've Just Met

What Ali MacGraw
Faces Now

Forgetting About
Orgasm—
The Best Way
to Have One!

Famous Diet Expert
Nathan Pritikin
Tells How to Diet
While Dining Out
(Without Dying
or Being a Bore)!

How to Have a Great
Bottom—What a
Girl Can Do
to Have a
Fair Derrière

Three Ways
(Without Them
Forget It)
to Make It Big

The Bishop
in the Back Seat,
Clarissa Watson's
Flashy, Funny
Mystery Thriller

Makeup by Way Bandy

Makeup artists we love... and lost

I can't write a chapter on makeup without mentioning a couple of the great artists who are no longer with us. The late, loved, and very-much-missed Way Bandy was a makeup artist who famously transformed many of the celebrated faces of the '70s and '80s. Way used his makeup like a sculptor, finding the bones, the hollows, the highlights, and making us look differently at the same faces we had become familiar with. After Way finished his handiwork, I hardly recognized the woman who gazed back at me from the mirror. He gave me cheekbones before I knew they were in there hiding! In Way's skilled hands, makeup was a powerful tool. We did many *Cosmo* covers together—I remember studying my face in the mirror, trying to figure out how he did it, before I had to wash his artistry down the drain.

I also had the great pleasure of working with the late Kevyn Aucoin. Kevyn had that special ability to see beauty and sculpt the canvas of the

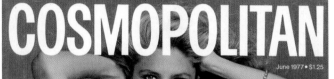

COSMOPOLITAN
June 1977 • $1.25

The Prime of
Mr. Gregory Peck

The Awful World
of a New Wife
Coping with
His Children
and How to
Keep Them from
Wrecking
the Marriage

Why Strong,
Terrific Girls
Get Hopelessly
Involved
with Losers

Sex and
the Formerly
Married

Legs Are Back—
and Gaining on
Bosoms—
How to Show
Yours Off
Outrageously

The Kept Woman
Is Alive and Well
(Sometimes) in This
Feminist Age—
Four Vivid
Case Histories

The Marilyn
Monroe Only
Her Hairdresser
Knew—an
Intimate Memoir

"End of a
Marriage?"
A Provocative
Excerpt from
Erica Jong's
Bell—Ringing
New Novel,
How to Save
Your Own Life

Plus James Brady's
Scarifying Thriller,
Paris One—
Low Doings in the
High Couture!

Makeup by Way Bandy

COSMOPOLITAN
December 1984 • $1.95

Is Your Bed
a Battlefield?
The Sexual
Power Game
Some Couples
Play

Everything
You Can Do Now
to Look
Desirable at 40

Why a Hot Young
Comedy Superstar
Is Wondering What
Life Is All About.
The Dark Side
of Bill Murray

Surviving Divorce
and Other
Emotional Disasters
That Shatter Your
Body and Mind

Life-Changing
Excerpt From
Leo Buscaglia's
Best-seller,
Loving
Each Other

Need to Lose
5 Pounds in a
Week? Follow
Cristina Ferrare's
Emergency Diet

A Man's View
of Women
Who Come On
Too Strong

Moving Up.
Ways to Advance
Your Career

Pages and Pages
of Christmas Cheer
and Carolyn Coker's
Cliff-hanging
Mystery Novel

Makeup by Sandy Linter
(who is, luckily, still with us)

face. As he worked, he'd tell me about overcoming the difficulties of growing up in the South as a gay man with a passionate interest in fashion and the art of makeup. But he remained true to his dreams and he found respect and success. That's the most important lesson. He was an artist who died too soon, but not before helping create indelible images of beauty, plus a great line of beauty products that bear his name. It was an honor to work with and learn from two such brilliant artists.

Our industry lost a lot of truly amazing people during the AIDS epidemic back in the '80s. It was a scary and sad time. I have a special place in my heart for two more sweethearts and major talents with whom I had the honor of working—Vincent Nasso and Bob Rule. Vincent was a brilliant makeup artist and a lot of fun. We traveled together for many shoots—my favorite was a trip to Saint Bart's for *Glamour* magazine. We had so much fun! From Vincent I learned about earth tones and orange-y,

glowing colors, as well as the importance of enjoying each precious moment of life we are blessed with. My most memorable trip with makeup artist Bob Rule was to Costa Careyes, Mexico, where we dressed up like pirates and painted masks right on our faces. He was brilliant and knew exactly how to apply only what was needed. He made everyone he touched feel beautiful—what a wonderful gift!

Everyday makeup for the active woman

Today's women are leading such busy, active lives that they need makeup that lasts through their very long to-do lists. I like to think of everyday makeup as your basic face—only better. It's about using the right products and techniques to define your features and cover any flaws, all with an almost imperceptible touch. Here are my step-by-step tips for putting on this basic face:

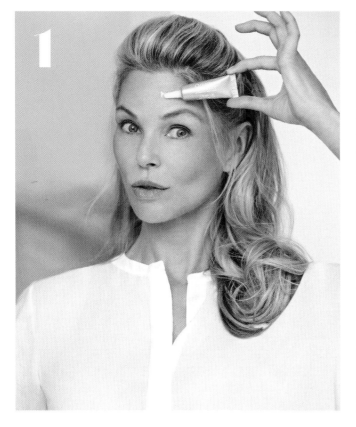

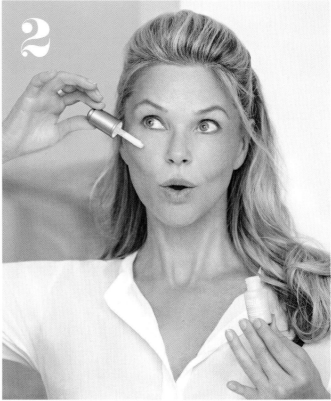

Start with my **Christie Brinkley Authentic Skincare CLOSE UP Instant Wrinkle Reducer & Treatment**. *I also like* **Chanel Le Blanc de Chanel Multi-Use Illuminating Base**.

Use **Christie Brinkley Authentic Skincare REFOCUS Eye + IR Defense** *under the eyes to protect and smooth that delicate skin.*

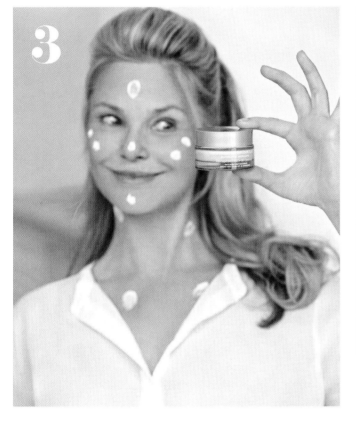

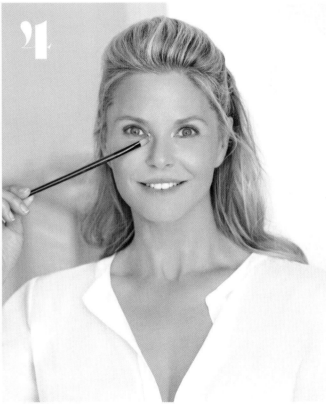

*Apply **Christie Brinkley Authentic Skincare RECAPTURE 360 + IR Defense Anti-Aging Day Cream** generously to your face and neck.*

*If I'm going to be at the beach or pool, I opt for a waterproof concealer, like **Kevyn Aucoin The Sensual Skin Enhancer** (in shade SX07). Apply it to the corner of the eye using a concealer brush, then blend (don't use your finger, because it will deposit too much and emphasize any fine lines). You can also smear some on the eyelid, stopping at the eye hollow crease. Set it with a fine dusting of powder to prevent the concealer from creasing in the folds of the eyelid.*

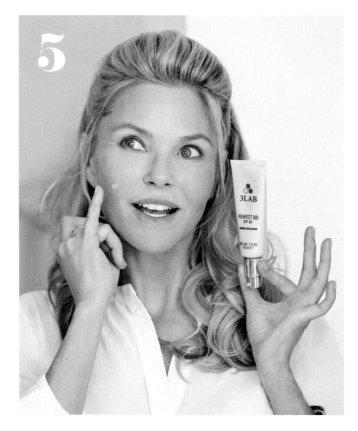

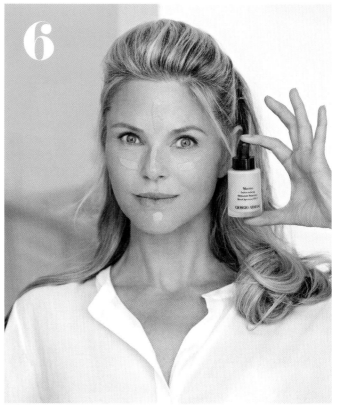

*Dot on, then blend in **3LAB Perfect BB Cream SPF 40**. This is a great way to add another layer of sun protection for a day outdoors—plus, it helps cover up hyperpigmented spots and even out skin tone. I use my fingers to blend and just go very lightly over any areas where I've applied concealer so that I don't rub that coverage off. Depending on your skin, you might not even need foundation over it.*

*If you want a a bit more coverage (that still lets your skin shine through), try **Giorgio Armani Maestro Octinoxate Sunscreen Fusion Makeup, Broad Spectrum SPF 15** (I use colors 6 and 7) and apply it using a **Kevyn Aucoin Foundation Brush**. The foundation is very sheer and liquid, so it's nearly undetectable in the light of day. I like to use the darker shade to carve out cheekbones and tie in my forehead. For the rest of my face I match my skin tone as closely as possible.*

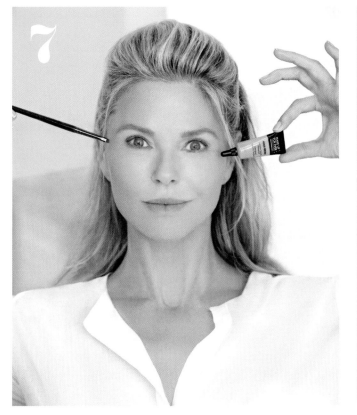

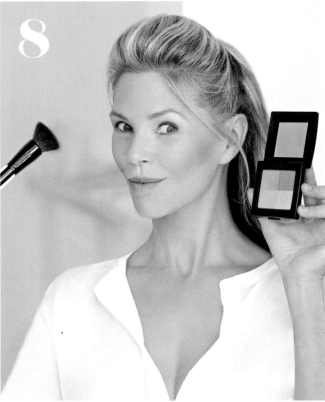

Define your brows with **Make Up For Ever Aqua Brow** *(I use color #10) using the* **Make Up For Ever Angled Eyebrow Brush no. 270**. *It will stay on all day (even if you go swimming!) so your face looks polished and defined—never washed out.*

I like to contour my face to add depth. **Laura Mercier Illuminating Powder in Mocha Spice Quad,** *applied with a* **Kevyn Aucoin Super Soft Buff Powder Brush,** *does the job perfectly.*

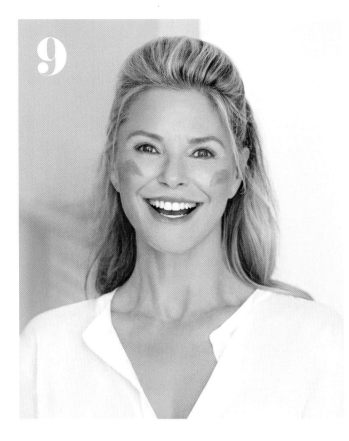

By Terry Hyaluronic Blush in #3 Bubble Glow *adds great, natural-looking color. Use the tiniest amount and blend it in immediately. You can use it for lips too—just add a dab to the center of your pout and use lip balm to smooth it out quickly.*

I like **Clarins Moisture Replenishing Lip Balm** *for colorless moisture.*

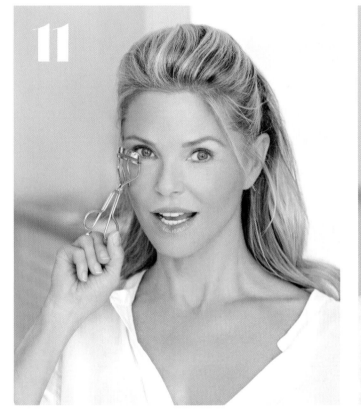

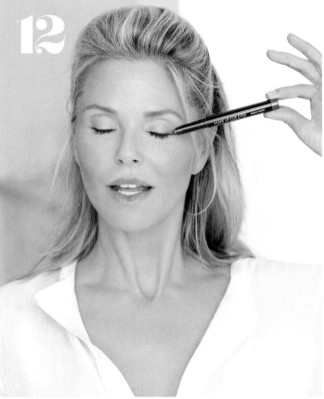

*Curl your lashes with **Kevyn Aucoin's The Eyelash Curler**. Never pull on your lashes, just get the curler down as close to your eyelid as you can without pinching or pulling and close it around your lashes. Do three little pumps, then release for the perfect curl.*

*Define eyes with **Make Up For Ever Aqua Matic Waterproof Glide-on Eye Shadow** (I use color S-60). I love this waterproof chubby pencil—use it in a back-and-forth motion along the base of the lashes until you have a defined line. (If you want to use a non-waterproof pencil, try **Lancôme Le Crayon Khôl in Black Ebony**.) I grab the skin at the outer corner of my eye and pull it toward my temple so that I'm stretching the skin flat and have a firmer edge to draw on.*

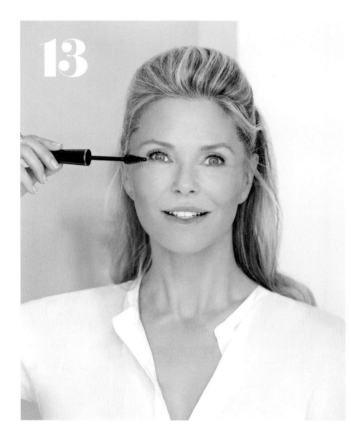

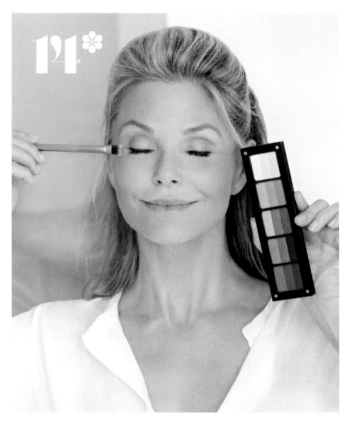

Add a coat of **Make Up For Ever Smoky Extravagant Mascara**. I like the wand because it goes from bushy on one end to tapered on the other so you can really get to the lashes in the inner corner.

A swipe of **Freedom System Eye Shadow in Orange** across the eyelids using a big fluffy brush will really emphasize blue eyes, and it's a warm, natural look for brown eyes too.

All together now

Here's everything I use in one handy place. Just go online (check the Resource Guide pages 195 and 196 for websites) and order them all for a brand-new you!

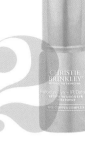

1 Christie Brinkley Authentic Skincare CLOSE UP Instant Wrinkle Reducer & Treatment

2 Christie Brinkley Authentic Skincare REFOCUS Eye + IR Defense

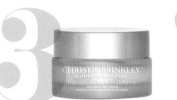

3 Christie Brinkley Authentic Skincare RECAPTURE 360 + IR Defense Anti-Aging Day Cream

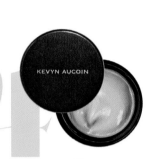

4 Kevyn Aucoin The Sensual Skin Enhancer

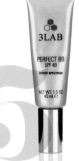

5 3LAB Perfect BB Cream SPF 40

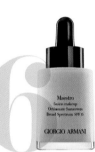

6 Giorgio Armani Maestro Octinoxate Sunscreen Fusion Makeup, Broad Spectrum SPF 15

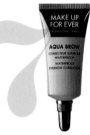

7 Make Up For Ever Aqua Brow

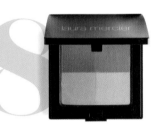

8 Laura Mercier Illuminating Powder in Mocha Spice Quad

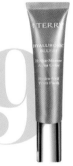

9 By Terry Hyaluronic Blush in #3 Bubble Glow

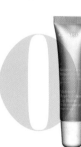

10 Clarins Moisture Replenishing Lip Balm

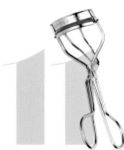

11 Kevyn Aucoin The Eyelash Curler

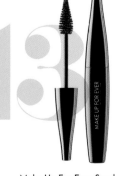

12 Make Up For Ever Aqua Matic Waterproof Glide-on Eye Shadow and Lancôme Le Crayon Khôl in Black Ebony

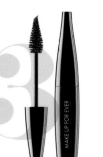

13 Make Up For Ever Smoky Extravagant Mascara

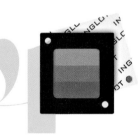

14 Freedom System Eye Shadow in Orange

Stepping it up to an office-worthy face

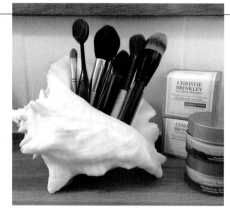

When you have a big meeting at work or an important interview, you might want a little extra polish (beyond the "basic" face you've just learned). Here's what I'd do differently:

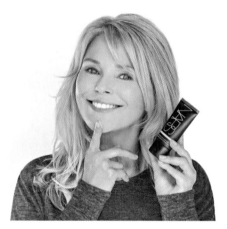

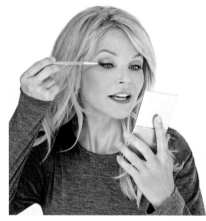

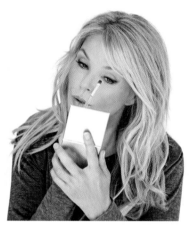

*Opt for a matte, long-lasting foundation (such as **NARS Sheer Matte Foundation** or **Bobbi Brown Long-Wear Even Finish Foundation**). Under harsh office lights, you'll want this extra coverage to make skin look flawless and polished. I often use two shades—the lighter one goes over my undereye concealer, then blends into the area above the cheekbone. I also put the lighter shade along the sides of my nose (along the marionette lines) and down along the jowls to brighten and lift a little. Then I'll use the darker shade under the cheeks and along the jaw to add contour and depth.*

For the eyes, do the same pencil liner, but extend it beyond the outer corner just a hint. Then take a tapered hard brush and use it to apply a warm, chocolate-brown powder to smudge along the lash line. You're adding more, but it actually has a softening effect.

*Neutral eye shadow works best for the office. I love the **Urban Decay Naked Basics Palette** to add contour and shape to the eyes. The colors are foolproof! (I use it with a **Sonia Kashuk for Target eye shadow brush**.)*

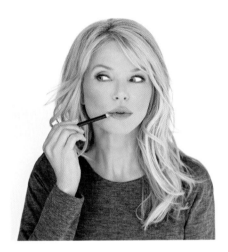

*Use a lip pencil (I like the ones by **Bobbi Brown**) to line and fill in your lips. The waxiness of the pencil will give your lipstick or gloss something to adhere to so it lasts longer (and if it does wear off, you won't be left with just a line around your lips!).*

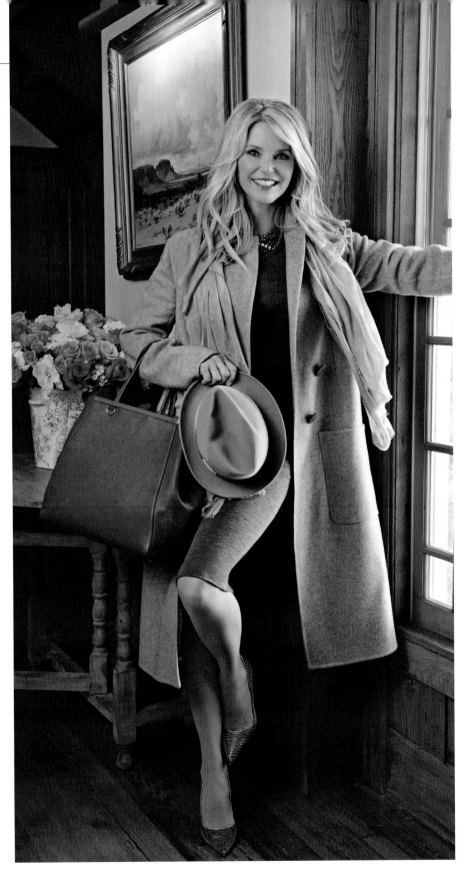

Turn your daytime makeup into an evening look

You don't have to start over from scratch before heading out to dinner. Taking your makeup up a notch is as simple as adding a little more definition and color to your face. Look, you can do it in just a few steps!

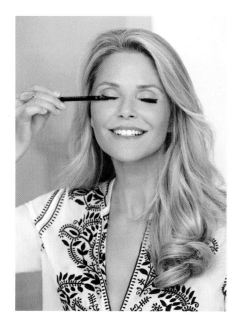 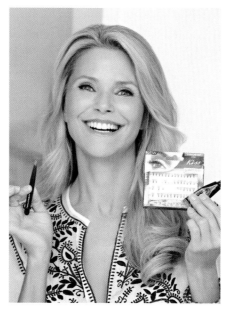 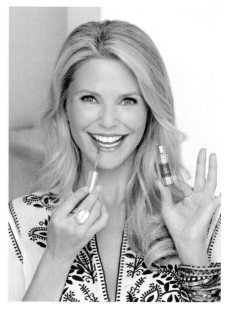

*Redefine eyes for a more dramatic evening look using **Make Up For Ever Aqua Eyes Eyeliner in color 25L**. Don't make one straight line; start at the inner corner of the eye with a thin line, then make it thicker at the outer corner of the eye. It's very important that the eyeliner gets tweaked up a bit at the outer corner—this helps you look awake and lifts the eye, especially important after a long day!*

*Adding some false lashes is a great way to give eyes even more oomph. I like **Kiss i-Envy Short Black Individual Lashes** applied with **Kiss Strip Lash Adhesive in Black**. Pick up the lashes with tweezers, dip in the adhesive, and apply directly to your lash line. And I LOVE their lash clumps for adding even more glamour!*

*You want your lips to look glossy all evening long. **Lancôme Lip Lover in color 356** is a beautiful red gloss that doesn't feather and has great staying power. I also love **NARS Lip Gloss in Sweet Dreams**— it's my go-to light pink shimmer. Apply the smallest amount you can get away with and it will stay forever—it's a funny paradox, but somehow less grips the lips better than more.*

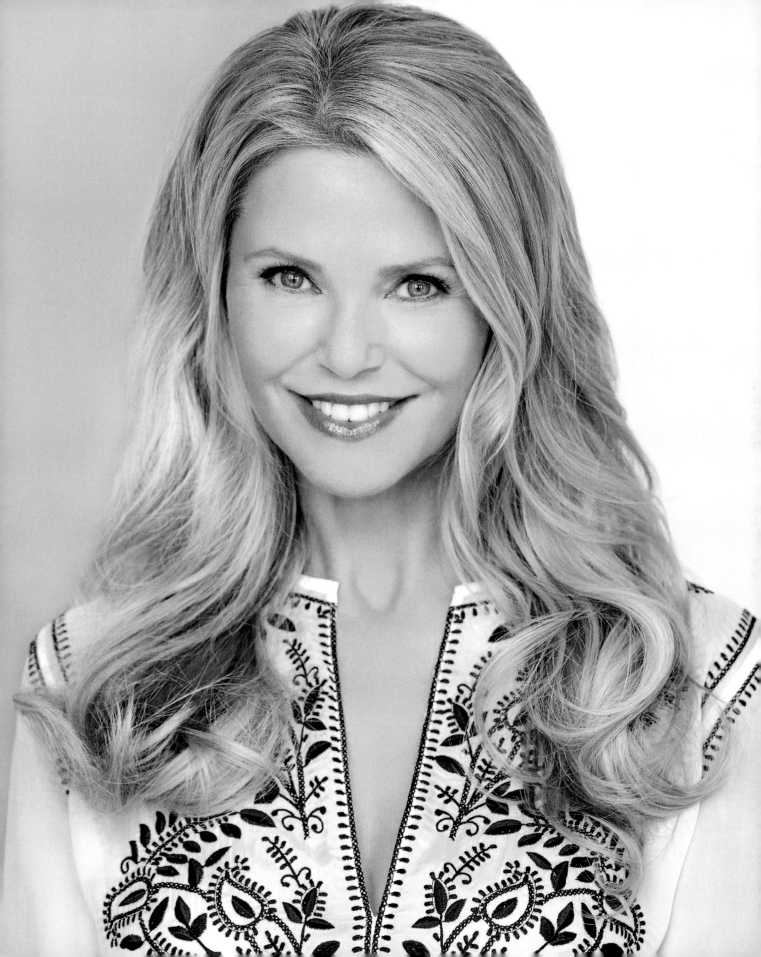

My twenty timeless makeup tips

Makeup, like fashion, changes every season. But certain shades and techniques will always work—and makeup that makes you look like you (only better) is always in style.

NUMBER
1

Always start with an exfoliator to make your skin feel smooth and flawless. Your foundation will glide on effortlessly, which will save you time in the long run! I use the creamy scrub from my **Authentic Skincare** line every morning. **St. Ives Fresh Skin Apricot Scrub** is a good alternative.

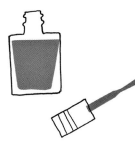

NUMBER
2

Do double duty with an antiaging moisturizer that has an SPF 30 broad-spectrum sunblock. Luckily today's moisturizers pack a lot of benefits in one bottle. I love my own **RECAPTURE 360 + IR Defense** and **Olay Regenerist Regenerating Lotion**.

NUMBER
3

Use a primer for added grip and smoothness. It'll help even out your skin tone by providing a consistent base for your foundation to adhere to, plus make foundation look fresher longer.

NUMBER
4

Choose your foundation so that the shade matches your skin perfectly at your jawline. That will make it quick and easy to blend all the edges—at your hairline and jaw—seamlessly.

NUMBER
5

Never try to use foundation to make you look tan (see my tips in chapter 4 about getting a fake glow).

NUMBER
6

Certain makeup shades are almost universally flattering. For day, it's brown, taupe, gray and bronze, pink and peach. At night, it's slate and black for more drama on the eyes.

NUMBER
7

Accentuate only one part of your face at a time. If you do a dark, dramatic eye, keep the lips pale. If you opt for bright lips, go easy on the eyes.

NUMBER
8

Blush should be the color your cheeks are after a run, or a really good compliment!

NUMBER
9

Don't overpluck your brows—you'll regret it later! They thin out naturally with age, so you'll want to define them for a more youthful look (read on in this chapter for specific how-tos).

NUMBER
10
Always check your makeup in different light sources—not just in your bathroom mirror. Check it by a window, near a lamp, or outside if you can.

NUMBER
11
If you're wearing a dress or top that is lower cut, throw a little of what's on your face on your collarbone and décolletage. Foundation, bronzer, blush—all will help make your face blend with your body so that it looks really natural. If you have sun spots on the backs of your hands, throw a touch on there too!

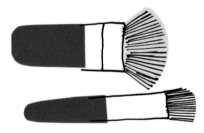

NUMBER
12
Use powder only in your T-zone, and use as little as possible.

NUMBER
13
Powder is to makeup what an eraser is to a pencil. You can use it on a puff to "erase" blotchy blush.

NUMBER
14
Don't use shimmery powder on wrinkles or any broken-out areas, because it will emphasize them.

NUMBER
15
Don't try to draw on lips that are larger than your own. Lip liner should stay inside the lines—it can be on the outer limits but should still be inside. Fill in the lips with pencil to save time making touch-ups later. And use a pencil and lipstick that match. (And remember, paler colors make lips look larger; darker ones make them look smaller.)

NUMBER
16
The lip color rule applies to other features as well. Pale concealer makes features seem larger and dark makes things recede. So don't use a concealer that's too light to try to hide undereye circles or a breakout, because it will have the opposite effect.

NUMBER
17
Spray **Evian** on your face after you've finished your makeup, then lay an open tissue on your face and pat over it to soak up the spray, taking with it that powdery look that can dull a glow!

NUMBER
18
To keep excess lipstick from ending up on your teeth, insert one finger into your mouth, close your just-lipsticked lips around your finger, and pull it out. The lipstick on your finger was destined for your teeth—all clear now!

NUMBER
19
When in doubt, less is more.

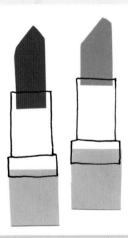

NUMBER
20
Smile!

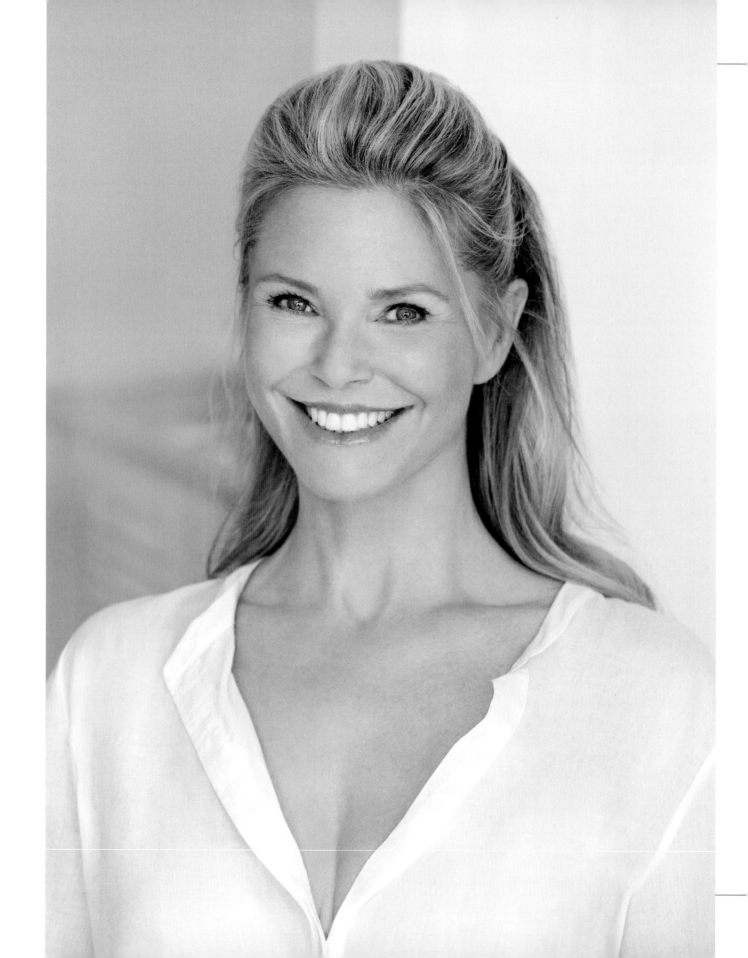

Brow know-how

Before you pick up the tweezers, wax, or even a brow pencil, there are a few eyebrow rules you should know—and follow—to make sure you don't raise any eyebrows in fear!

Step back and look at your brows in the context of your whole face several times while tweezing your brows. It's easy to get obsessed with the small picture and carried away with the tweezers when you're up against the magnifying mirror.

"Your brows need to last you a lifetime, so treat them with respect!" says makeup artist Sandy Linter (and I agree!).

Don't ever tweeze above the brows. As you age, your brows will start to sag a bit, so plucking them from underneath will create a subtle, flattering arch.

The shape of your brows can speak volumes. Bringing them too close together will make you look like you're scowling. Extending out and down on the outside edges will make you look sad.

Every makeup artist will have a different favorite trick, but for novices, brow powder may be more forgiving than pencil for filling in and defining brows. "Powder goes on lighter and more natural looking, while pencil can look too solid and heavy," says makeup artist Denise Markey.

I look at the deepest shade in my hair and accent that. I start by applying a darker brown very lightly along the middle to upper part of my brows, then switch to a lighter one and feather it out to the sides. It gives me more volume and looks the most natural.

Use an extra-large eyebrow brush to soften and blend powder and pencil. It's also great for dabbing some eye shadow on your hairline to disguise roots or thin spots.

"I like to say that your eyebrows are 'sisters, not twins,'" says Linter. In other words, they shouldn't look identical. So don't try to tweeze one to totally match the other. "Treating them individually gives the face more character," says Linter.

My eyebrow best bets

I use **Laura Mercier Brow Powder in Deep Blonde** for everyday. If I do a darker eye or if I want a stronger, fuller brow, I add a **Laura Mercier** pencil in the same shade—making tiny strokes in the same direction as the hair growth. For a really dramatic brow, I turn to **Chanel Le Sourcil de Chanel**. The compact contains three powders—from taupe to dark brown. I put the deepest color down the middle of my brow and then edge it with the other two colors. It creates a full but very natural-looking brow. I also love **Lancôme Le Crayon Poudre** pencils in **Sable** and **Natural Blonde**. My latest favorite brow product is **Giorgio Armani Eye & Brow Maestro**. It contains a gel-like powder that is both eye shadow and eyebrow definer. It's fast and easy to use and comes in a lot of colors—I am having fun experimenting with them!

Anti-aging secrets

The right makeup can take years off your face. (And the wrong makeup can add extra years!) The trick is knowing which formulas, colors, and techniques will give you that youthful boost. It's all about accentuating the positive and eliminating the negative!

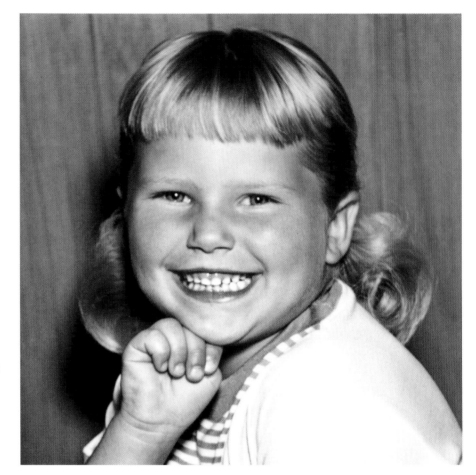

CONCEALER: Undereye concealer is a great tool for covering dark circles, but the older you get, the more sparing you want to be with it. You think you're concealing by caking it on, but really you're exposing every wrinkle you have around your eyes! I find using two colors—a lighter one in the inner and outer corners and darker to blend—works best. Also, know when to use your fingers or a brush—and that depends on the product. I use my fingers to do the darker part so that my body heat helps melt them together. It's almost magical how it conceals! Once I'm satisfied with the coverage, I only powder it lightly.

DEFINE: Add color to define cheeks, jawline, décolletage, hands. Too-pale shades or a monochromatic look is hard to pull off as you get older. Instead, try warm shades of blush to liven up your complexion. I like mixing two powder blushes together—one in a bronze tone and one that's more pink—and sometimes I pat a shimmery cream on top to reflect light and get that dewy look that's incredibly youthful.

LASHES: It's a fact that as you get older you start to lose hair (don't you hate that fact?), and unfortunately, that includes your eyelashes. So for an evening out or for photographs, I may add a few false lashes. There are so many options now, from single lashes to clumps of four lashes, plus strips in every length and fullness, so you can really choose to be as natural or as dramatic as you want! They are so easy to use and the result looks so fun and flirty and perfectly polished, yet natural. I am partial to black lashes, and I look for a short length, but I almost always also trim them down, both to fit horizontally and shorter so they don't look overdone. With individuals or clumps, I always use tweezers to pull them from the box and place them along my lash line. I start at the outside and

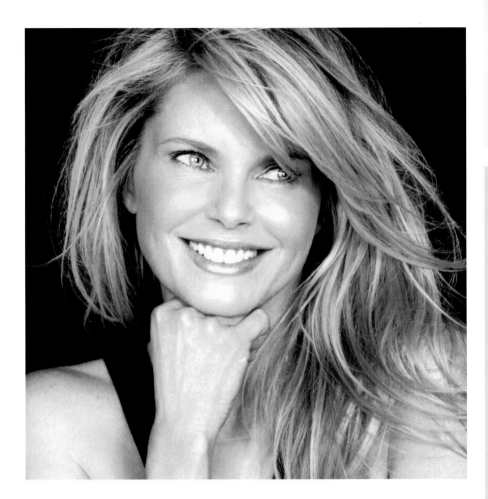

SPONGES!

The best makeup sponges are by **Alcone**. And makeup artist Sandy Linter taught me a great trick—if you have too much foundation on your face, use a dampened makeup sponge to bring it down till it looks more natural.

CUSTOM PALETTES

I love palettes—they're such an easy way to organize several makeup shades together. **Bobbi Brown**'s customizable palettes are great because you can put together your favorite color eye shadows and blushes all in one easy-access, mirrored case. I have two of the six-pan palettes—one filled with all blacks and grays and one filled with all taupes and browns. Perfect for traveling!

Inglot Cosmetics Freedom System palettes for face, lips, eyes, and blush come in a huge variety of colors. And makeup artists are often packing several **Viseart** palettes. I love the one for lips!

work in. Don't use any in the inner corner of the eye or it can make your eyes look too close together. I like to use mascara before I apply them—it gives the lashes a little more to grab on to—and then afterward, just sweep one coat onto the outer corners to sort of seal them together. If I use a whole lash, I trim it from the outer corner to fit my eye perfectly. I use a magnifying mirror to set it as close to my real lashes as possible, starting at the inner corner. I pinch it together with my own lashes with flat-edged tweezers. (And I always carry glue with me when I wear them, because you never know when something is going to make you cry!)

LIPS: I love **NARS Sweet Dreams**, a shimmery pale pink lip gloss, for everyday, used with **Spice** lip liner by **MAC**. That combo helps make lips look fuller, and that definitely makes you look younger! I also love a kind of bougainvillea pink lip because it just looks happy. And everyone needs to find their perfect red because it's classic and, yes, timeless!

EYE TOUCH-UP

I always keep **YSL Touche Éclat** in my bag to touch up that little dark spot at the inner corners of my eyes. As soon as the darkness bleeds through, I look instantly tired, but when I dab this on, it immediately wakes up my face. But I don't apply it straight from the brush that's built into the tube. I dab it onto my finger first and work off that.

MEET THE MAKEUP ARTIST:
Sandy Linter

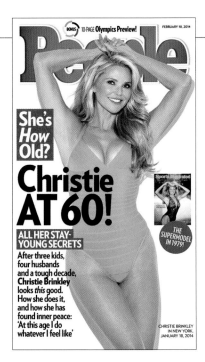

I think it was on a shoot for *Vogue* in 1975 in Florida when I first met Sandy. I remember she painted my face as though she'd been doing it her whole life—probably because we have the same coloring. I remember thinking, *What a funny and cool New Yorker!* Forty (!) years and hundreds of photographs later, we're both still doing what we love. I love working with Sandy. She's a true professional who will tell you why she's using which brush and share new products, so you get a look, a lesson, and a new way of looking at yourself, which is always refreshing.

"The first time I worked with Christie I couldn't believe how beautiful her skin coloring was. It's a makeup artist's dream to work on skin like that! I also loved her face shape—square jawline, high cheekbones. Her face absolutely popped from the page. I knew right away this was a model I wanted to work with again (and again and again, it turns out!). As a makeup artist, she really inspired me. I think my favorite jobs we did together were our numerous covers with the photographer Francesco Scavullo. I loved working with the two of them together. And the results were always so beautiful."

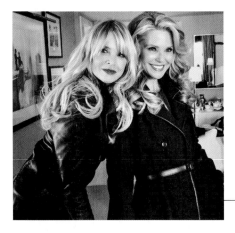

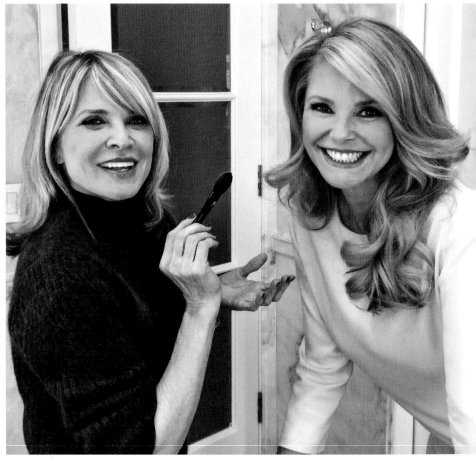

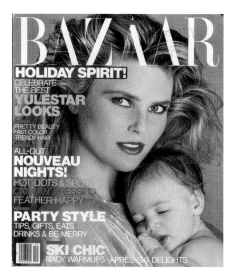

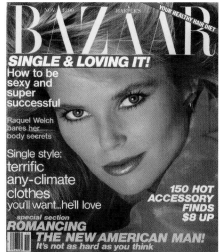

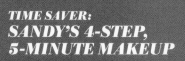

MASTER CLASS WITH SANDY

"I work in the reverse order of what I think a lot of women do when they apply their own makeup. I start with the eyes, then clean up any smudged liner or shadow with a little moisturizer on a Q-tip, then apply foundation, then cheek color, and concealer last. The reason I do the concealer last is that—especially as you age—you want to use as little as possible.

"A dot of highlighter (like **Yves Saint Laurent Touche Éclat**) right in the indentation at the inner corner of the eyes really opens them up and helps brighten the whole eye area.

"Don't use a concealer that's too light under your eyes or the result will look ashen. If you can't completely camouflage dark circles, divert attention away from them by curling the lashes and using liner to help lift the outer corner of the eye.

"Always use primer on your eyelids to keep your shadow and liner looking fresh all day.

"To give eyes a lift, stop your liner right at the outer corner and blend your shadow upward. To make eyes look wider, extend the line just beyond the outer edge.

"Too much powder can be aging. Dewy skin looks much more youthful."

QUICK TIP
KEEP YOUR EYELASH CURLER CLEAN!

Those little rubber strips in your eyelash curler can get gunked up with mascara. And if you don't clean them off regularly, your lashes could stick to the curler and get snapped off. When the rubber starts to wear out (or doesn't come clean), replace them.

TIME SAVER:
SANDY'S 4-STEP, 5-MINUTE MAKEUP

Try this quick, bare-bones routine when you need to get out the door—looking fresh-faced and polished—in no time flat!

1. ADD CONCEALER JUST WHERE YOU NEED IT MOST—ESPECIALLY AT THE INNER CORNER OF THE EYE. LINTER LOVES **LANCÔME LE CORRECTOR PRO CONCEALER KIT.** IT PUTS TWO SHADES OF CONCEALER, A FINISHING POWDER, AND A BRUSH IN ONE PALETTE.

2. DUST SOME BRONZER OVER YOUR CHEEKS AND ANYWHERE ELSE YOU NEED A LITTLE COLOR.

3. USE AN EYE PENCIL TO LINE YOUR EYES AND UNDER THE EYE TO ADD DEFINITION.

4. APPLY A LIP GLOSS.

You're ready to go!

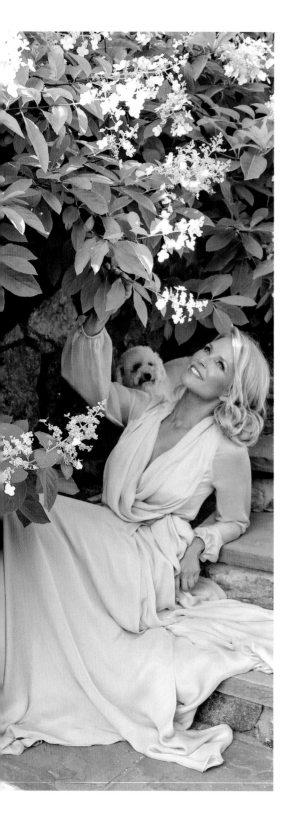

WATCH THE WEATHER

Pay attention to the condition of your skin—and the weather report—when prepping your face for makeup. During the winter or when I'm in a really dry climate, I add plenty of moisture to my skin before I apply anything else. I might even switch to a richer formula of foundation and a creamier blush. But if I took that same approach on a hot, humid day, my makeup would literally slide right off my face! That's when I reach for an oil-free primer, a lighter, less emollient foundation, and powder blushes. (I was once on a red carpet when all of a sudden, in front of a million paparazzi, my makeup started to drip right off onto the red carpet! I was using a product that contained a humectant, which attracts moisture from the air, and on that warm, humid evening it attracted a little too much moisture!)

TIME TO
MULTI-TASKERCISE!

While you're sorting through your beauty products and throwing away old makeup that has expired (especially important for mascara), sneak in some more "multi-taskercises." Stand on one leg and do twenty calf raises—rising slowly up and down on your toes. Then switch sides and do the same on the other leg. Keep going till your calves can really feel it—you need strong calves to rock your Manolos and sexy Brian Atwoods!

QUICK TIP
INNER BEAUTY

Now that you've perfected your curb appeal, check out the last chapter in this book for information on ways to share your good fortune and give back to the world to buff up your inner beauty! One organization that literally makes me smile just thinking of the lives they change is Smile Train. They offer life-altering surgery to children born with a cleft palate whose families could otherwise never afford to pay for it. They also teach local doctors to perform the surgeries so they can continue to help long after Smile Train has moved on to help other children. The smile on the child's face is surpassed only by the smiles on the parents' faces when they see their son or daughter healed for the first time.

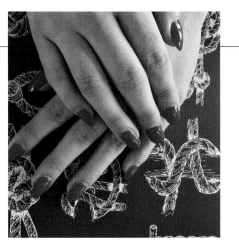

Nailing it in no time!

Tips for sleek hands and feet

I don't have the time or patience to sit still for a salon manicure and pedicure. But I still like my nails to look nice. Here are a few tricks I've picked up from manicurists I've met on shoots—and that I use to keep my hands and feet looking polished (literally!).

When nails get stained or look yellow from wearing dark polish, rub a little tea tree oil onto them. Do it every day and soon they'll return to their natural, healthy color. (A solution of half distilled white vinegar and half water works too.)

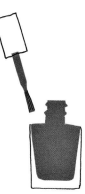

Vicks VapoRub can help fight fungal infections—just work a dab underneath your nails. Or soak your nails in a bowl of apple cider vinegar.

Dr. Gendler's Foot Recovery Cream can soften even an old surfer's foot cracked from the salt and sea (like mine!). **Dermasil** lotion is another good option for keeping hands and feet soft.

I recently started taking **BioSil**—it's a hair, nail, and skin vitamin. It makes my nails grow visibly faster!

For toes, always cut or file nails straight across to prevent ingrown nails. For fingers, I still follow the rule my mom taught me, which is to file the nails so that the shape mimics that of the half-moon at the base of your nails.

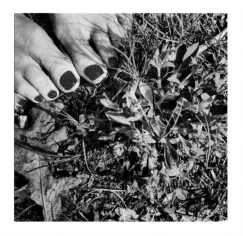

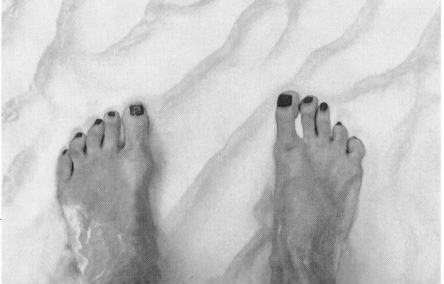

MEET THE MAKEUP ARTIST:
Denise Markey

I think the most exciting job I ever did with Denise was my billboard in Times Square for *Chicago the Musical*. The photo was done while I was still in rehearsals for the show and I was still trying to figure out my character, Roxie Hart. Denise gave me the perfect Roxie face—with the smoky eyes and Roxie red lips done to such perfection that they even looked great on a billboard several stories high! She really can do anything from very natural to the demands of TV lighting. All with a sweet smile and a sharp eye making sure everything is perfect for the shot.

"I was so nervous the first time I worked with Christie. After all, she is such a beauty icon! But she was so warm, welcoming, and gracious that I quickly forgot to be nervous and we had a great day. She is truly an inspiring woman. And every time that I've had the pleasure of working with her, her positive attitude is infectious. I believe that this great attitude is the quality that makes Christie one of the most beautiful women in the world!"

MASTER CLASS WITH DENISE

"I love using a concealer palette. My favorite is the **Kryolan Dermacolor Mini Concealer Palette** from **Alcone**. It'll take a little trial and error to figure out which combinations of shades work, but you'll have all the colors you need to conceal under-eye circles, blemishes, dark spots, bruises." (Denise has me hooked on these palettes. They're great when you just want to cover where you need it and not put foundation on the whole face.)

"Start with a shade that's lighter than your skin tone to cover up darkness, and then add a layer of a darker color (that's a closer match to the rest of your skin) so that it blends seamlessly. This technique will make hyperpigmented spots vanish.

"Skip the powder brush and use a fine sponge instead when applying powder after your foundation. I find that a sponge lays down a finer veil of powder that blends seamlessly with the foundation, while a brush dusts the surface and does not set the foundation as well.

"If you're getting your picture taken (or even think you might snap a selfie), skip or go very lightly on anything that has a lot of pearl or frost to it. The camera flash reflects and exaggerates the frost and can make the face look too shiny.

"I use the **Light** or **Medium Clarifier** eye pencil from **Three Custom Color** to line the inside of the lower eyelids. It makes the whites of the eyes look bigger and brighter."

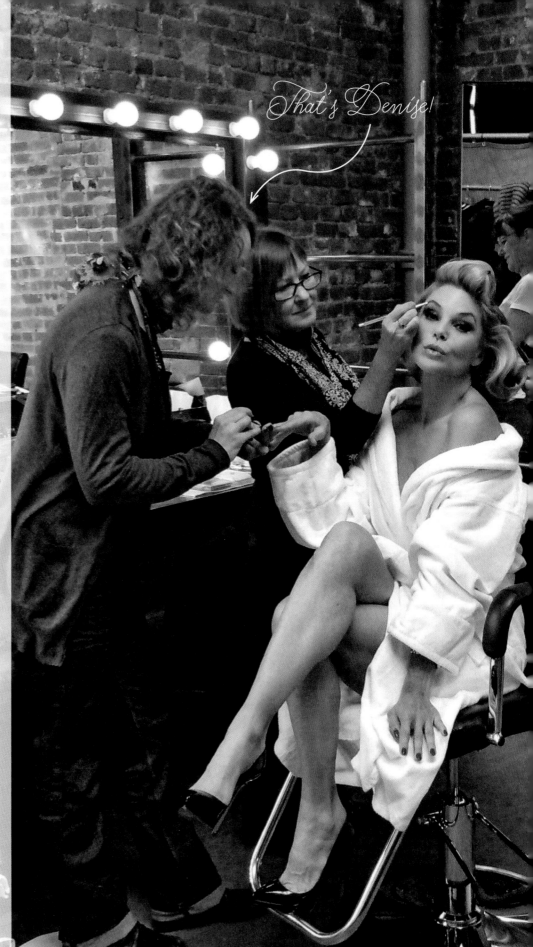

" What makes someone truly beautiful is being beautiful on the inside. That radiates through and makes you glow—like no makeup can! "

—Denise

That's Denise!

MEET THE MAKEUP ARTIST:
Moyra Mulholland

Moyra is an incredible painter. I guess I shouldn't have been surprised after all the famous faces she has painted! But Moyra also paints canvas and, in my opinion, her talent is on par with the perfectionistic brush-strokes of Andrew Wyeth. And she brings that same level of detail to her makeup. She's also a bit of a scientist—always reading about ingredients and mixing and playing around with products. I remember the first time I worked with her, I thought she was the other model. I was so surprised when she took out her brushes and started painting my face! Brains and beauty, that's Moyra.

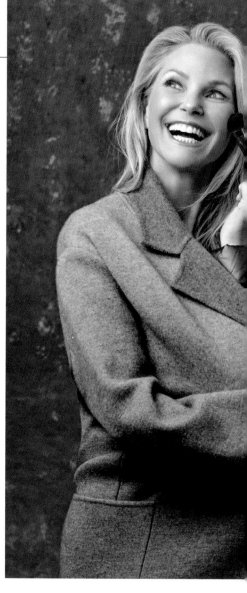

"My first job with Christie was a photo shoot for *Harper's Bazaar* at her house on the beach, probably about twenty-five years ago. I remember that her daughter Alexa was just a tiny tot. I was still new to the scene so feeling a bit nervous to be working with Christie Brinkley! I was a little bit in awe, but she has an amazing way of making everyone feel totally at ease. She's also incredibly funny. Every time we work together there is so much laughter."

MASTER CLASS WITH MOYRA

"When I'm doing my own makeup, I mix together some moisturizer, sunscreen, and a primer that has some reflective particles and then rub it all over my face with my hands. It helps to even everything out so that you only need to add foundation or concealer in spots.

"Hyaluronic acid attracts water to the skin. So I use a hyaluronic acid gel—sometimes mixed with a little foundation—to make the skin look dewy. Skip it when the weather's humid, though.

"The secret to foundation that really lasts all day is adding water on top of it (after foundation and powder have been applied). It's an old theater trick. I dampen a sponge with a spray bottle of **Evian** and just pat the face like that. Then I very gently pat it with a flat piece of tissue. It'll help remove excess that can leave the skin looking powdery and restore a dewiness to the skin." (Yes! I've been doing this ever since Moyra taught me this trick—it really does bring out the skin's glow.)

"I use a regular graphite art pencil instead of a brow pencil. I like it better because you can really simulate the look of hair without leaving any residue stuck in your brows. I use a harder one on blondes, a slightly softer one on darker brows.

"Applying mascara is the single most important thing you can do to change your face. I never skip this step. It really opens up the eyes.

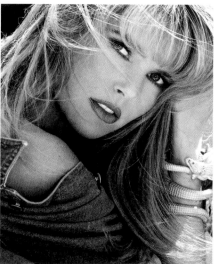

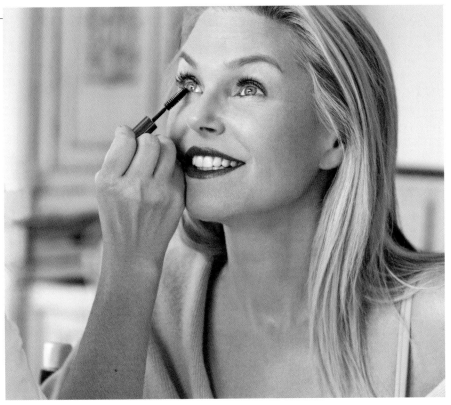

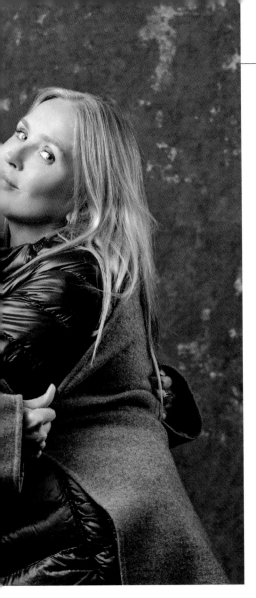

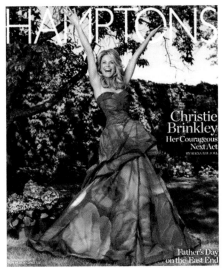

"The newer liquid liners are so easy to use, really almost foolproof. I like **Physicians Formula Eye Booster 2-in-1 Lash Boosting Eyeliner + Serum**. Draw a fine line just on the outer quarter of the upper lash line, extending it just slightly beyond the eye.

"I like to pick a really intense shade of blush—the kind of color you'd look at and think, 'Oh no, I can't put that on my face!' Then put it on and rub really hard, almost buffing it into the skin with the brush. That way, you deposit the pure, long-lasting pigment directly into the foundation you've applied.

"Don't make your foundation and powder an exact match—to each other or to your skin tone. It will look too mask-like. I like to use a slightly deeper yellow foundation with a pinkish powder on top to give more depth to the skin.

"I love the idea of lipstick, but I feel like it often looks too harsh and fake. So I mix up a dark stain of color and use that. I'll take a little dab of **DuWop Lip Venom** and mix colors into it. You could use a dab of lipstick, some powdered eye shadow, or blush—just play with it until you come up with a shade you like. Sometimes I'll add a tiny bit of gold for some shimmer. I apply it with a lip brush and then take my finger, dip it into foundation, and pat it over the lips to take the color back a bit and give it staying power."

See what I mean? Moyra really is part scientist, part artist!

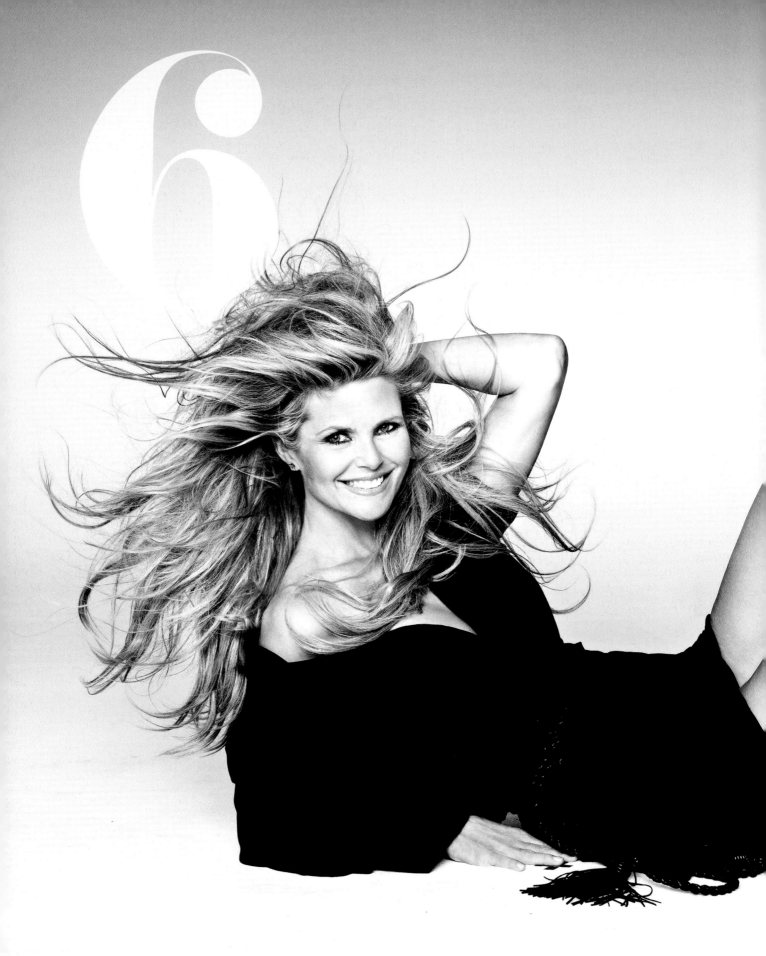

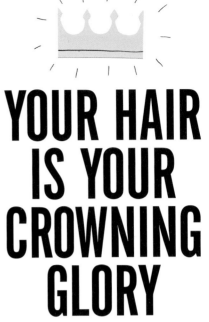

YOUR HAIR IS YOUR CROWNING GLORY

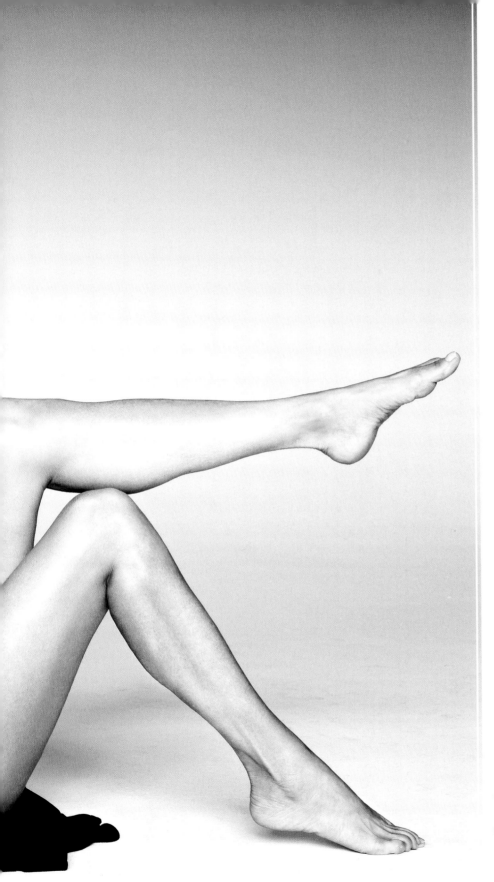

Let your hair down, and watch your spirits go up!

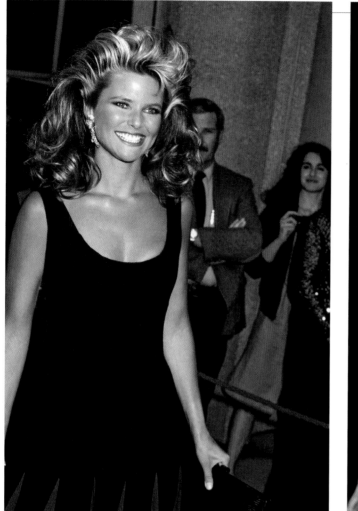

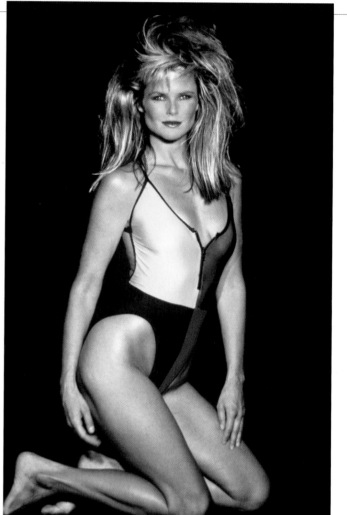

Let's face it. Everything is better on a good hair day. You can get away with anything—the wrong outfit, shoes, job— none of it matters as much when your hair looks good! Because when your hair looks great, you feel great. And that confidence makes you look even more attractive!

I've always been a bit obsessed with hair. Even when I was little, if I heard my mom say I was going to have my picture taken, I would immediately grab the scissors and "trim" my own bangs. All my childhood photos are of me grinning from ear to ear with my way-too-short bangs chopped right down to the scalp!

And long before I actually became a model, I loved to dress up, do "high-fashion hairdos," and strike poses.

Then when I became a model, nobody would let me cut my hair. The shortest I ever had it was just above the shoulders. I was trying to channel Grace Kelly, but to no avail—short hair is a lot of work! During my years as a model, my hair was often under contract. I've been a Breck girl (classic shampoo!) and a longtime Prell girl (if your hair ever feels bogged down with product, just one shampoo with Prell and your hair will be light and full and shiny). And I even made a few appearances on Clairol

boxes. During my forty-year career, I learned so much about hair that when I had my three kids, I became their personal hairdresser for haircuts and styling! I even did the hair for many of my daughter Alexa's shows.

I've worn my hair long nearly all my life, and at sixty, I see no reason to change that. Thankfully, gone are the days when long hair was considered "inappropriate" for a woman past a certain age (and I believe that age was about thirty!). I say if you've got long hair that works for you, there's no reason not to keep working it.

Over the years, I've put my hair

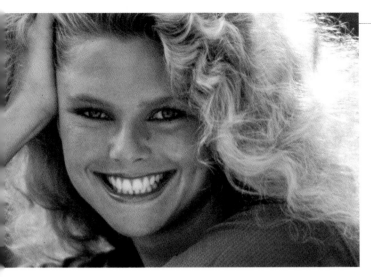

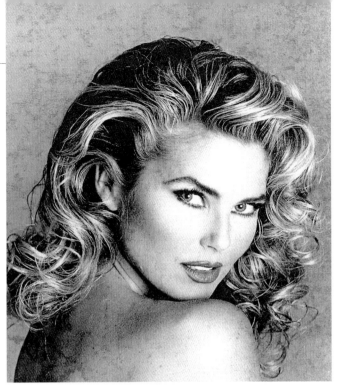

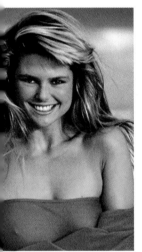

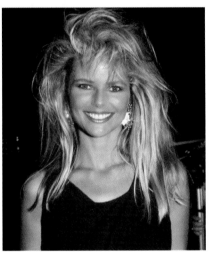

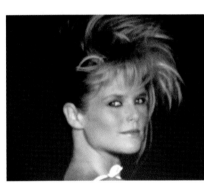

Some of my hairdos over the years

in the hands of many talented professionals for photo shoots and red carpet events. And I love all the opportunities I have had to learn from them. They are at photo shoots all the time, so they know the latest trends to help keep me looking modern and up-to-date. So between all my own trial-and-error expertise and the knowledge I've gleaned from my favorite hairstylists, I've got lots of shortcuts and tips to share. And I promise they'll make your hair your "mane" attraction and improve your chances of making every day a great hair day!

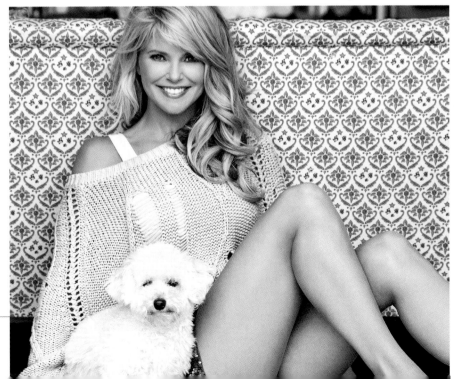

Nutrition is the "root" of gorgeous hair

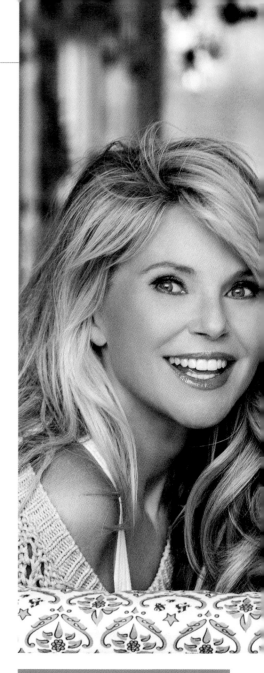

Just like for your skin, the right foods and supplements really can make a difference when it comes to your hair. Without a balanced diet, hair can thin, get brittle, and lose its luster.

Amino acids are the building blocks of healthy hair. There are twenty amino acids, but nine of them are considered essential—meaning the body can't make them, so you must get them in your diet. Essential amino acids are found in foods that contain protein. It's easy to get all your essential amino acids from animal foods like meat, poultry, seafood, eggs, and dairy. You can also get your amino acids through a vegetarian diet, but only a few plant foods contain all nine essential amino acids (nutritional superstars like quinoa, soybeans, and hemp seeds). If you are vegetarian or vegan, it's a good idea to take an amino acid supplement to ensure you get adequate amounts.

Several different amino acids are crucial for hair. Methionine forms sulfur chains that strengthen the structure of the hair and protect against hair loss. A study found that people taking methio-

nine had a higher percentage of hair in the growth phase—and that translates to more hair growing in, less falling out, and a thicker head of hair! Arginine improves blood flow to the hair follicles to nourish hair as it grows. And glutamine (which is produced naturally by the body, but diminishes as we get older) also delivers hair-building sulfur to your strands.

You also want to make sure you're feeding your hair plenty of B vitamins and zinc—through either diet or supplements. I take extra B vitamins because those nutrients are also predominantly found in animal foods, so it's really tough for vegetarians to get enough of them. You'll know if you're deficient in Bs if your hair gets dull and brittle. Zinc is essential for building both keratin (the protein hair is made of) and collagen. And while we mostly think of collagen as the substance that keeps skin looking smooth, young, and wrinkle-free, it also contributes to a healthy scalp that can hold on to hair better. Foods high in zinc include oysters, shrimp, grass-fed beef, lentils, sesame seeds, and pumpkin seeds.

QUICK TIP
FIND THE SWEET SPOT

I've been told by numerous hairstylists that there is one universally flattering place for a ponytail—the spot on the back of your head that's on the same level as your nose. Put it there, and it's like getting an instant face-lift.

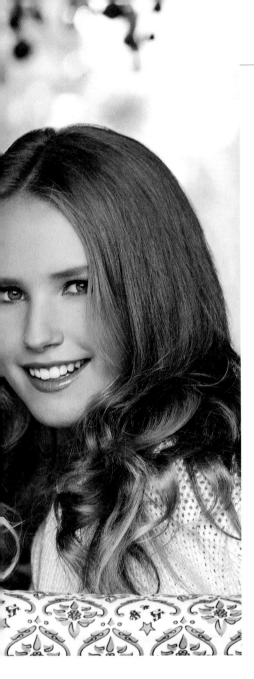

Don't lose your head over thinning hair

How you eat can also have a huge impact on how full your head of hair looks. Being deficient in iron or vitamin D can lead to hair loss (your doctor can do a blood test to check both). Vitamin D is produced by the body when our skin is exposed to sunlight, but our vigilant use of sunscreen—plus increased air pollution—can keep us from getting that boost. You'll also find D in fortified foods like milk and breakfast cereal. If you're deficient, supplements will probably be your best bet. Crash dieting of any kind can leave your hair follicles without the nutrients they need to generate healthy, new hair. So that's yet another reason to stop "deny-iting"!

While most women don't technically go bald in the same way men do, by a certain age, most of us do start to notice that making our hair look great just isn't that easy anymore. I know that for me, after each of my pregnancies my ponytail got just a little bit smaller. (And then my children became teenagers and I nearly pulled the rest out! LOL!) Some women do suffer from hereditary hair loss, and the hormonal changes that accompany menopause can make the

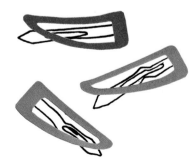

problem worse. An over- or underactive thyroid can also be a culprit—as can polycystic ovarian syndrome—so getting those things checked out by a doctor is a good idea if you're suddenly seeing significantly more strands than usual in the shower drain.

I've learned that as we age, not only is it natural to lose a few more strands, but the new strands grow in smaller and finer than they once did. Keeping your scalp healthy and your follicles well nourished can help. Do a quickie scalp massage every time you wash your hair to increase circulation. And consider doing an occasional antiaging scalp treatment—a leave-in mask that delivers important nutrients directly into the hair follicles.

Finally, if hair loss is becoming a big deal, you should see your dermatologist. There are numerous treatments doctors can use to help—from prescribing minoxidil (also available over the counter as **Rogaine**) to doing a variety of procedures that have been shown to help regrow hair, including lasers, cortisone injections, and platelet-rich plasma injections.

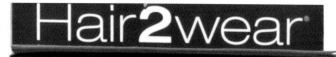

Model hair, no matter what!

Hair extensions have been a staple in the fashion and beauty worlds—as well as in Hollywood—forever. Models on the runway and stars on the red carpet routinely add extra strands to gain some length, thickness, or just enhance their glamour quotient. Today it seems like everybody's onto the convenience and style boost extensions can give. I love them so much that I collaborated on my own line of extensions by **Hair2wear**. Longer, thicker hair will always look youthful, so popping in an extension is my favorite quick and easy way to look years younger. Hair extensions allow you to change your hair as easily as you'd change your outfit. I like to think of them as the hairstyle equivalent of a microwave dinner. There are some days you feel like cooking, and some days you just want to pop something in the microwave. Definitely don't save extensions just for special occasions—I use mine at the gym, on rainy days, after the beach—they're perfect for anyone who wants to look great in an instant!

My hair extension how-tos

A long extension piece is an incredibly versatile hair accessory. As long as you have shoulder-length or longer hair yourself—ideally, the piece shouldn't extend more than four inches beyond your natural hair at the bottom—you can use it for a variety of styles. If I place it closer to the crown of my head, it adds tremendous volume. If I place it down lower, it adds volume, plus some extra length. And if you have the time after you get the extension in, use your curling iron or flat iron to style your own hair to add a wave or two near your face to match the extension's waves. It's the finishing touch that really makes it look seamless and perfect! Here's how to add one in a snap:

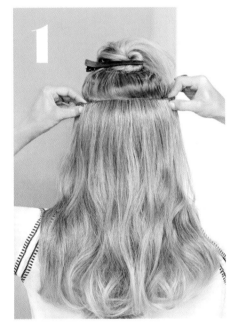 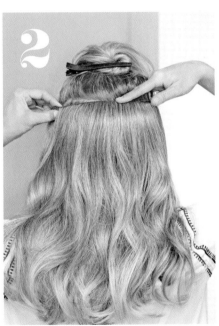 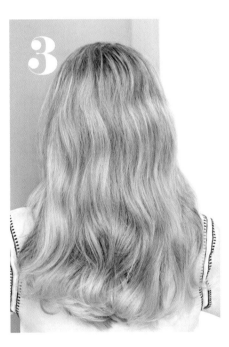

Hair2wear extensions come with a clip to pin the top portion of your hair up and hold it there while you position the extension. If you have fine, slippery hair, you may want to back-comb some hair at the area where you will clip. Hair spray or thickening spray on the clipping spots will also help increase the hair's grip.

I usually clip the ends and then do the middle clip straight across. But if you want to add length, add the clips slightly lower and drop the middle clip down (so that the extension is shaped like a smile) before clipping.

Voilà! You're done. But if your hair is stick-straight, use a medium- or-large-barrel curling iron on your own hair only—on either side and on top.

Caring for your hair extensions

Like your real hair, your extensions need a little TLC. Here are some of my favorite tricks for keeping them looking great:

• After you've worn your extensions a few times, you may want to wash them. It's easy: I like to mix in a tiny bit of dish soap with the shampoo—it gives the hair a really great shine.

• Lay the extension flat on a towel to dry. The built-in curls will come right back when it's dry. If you want to change the style by using a blow-dryer, curling iron, or flat iron, make sure to use it on the lowest setting to avoid burning or damaging the strands.

• If your hair is shoulder length or shorter, it's a good idea to take your extensions with you when you go see your hairstylist. She can trim the ends to make them blend more naturally into your own hair. And the layers can be trimmed to flatter your face shape.

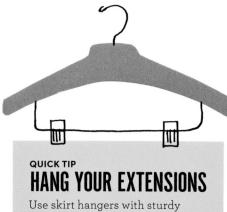

QUICK TIP
HANG YOUR EXTENSIONS
Use skirt hangers with sturdy clips to hang your extensions. It's a great way to organize them for styling and for storing.

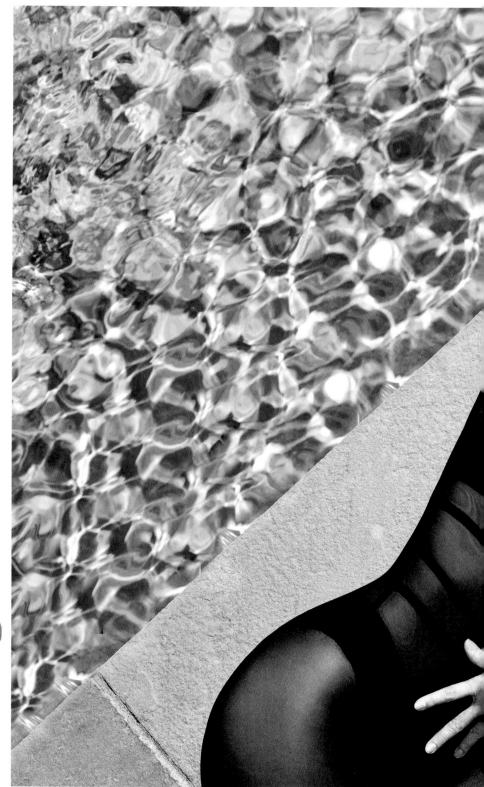

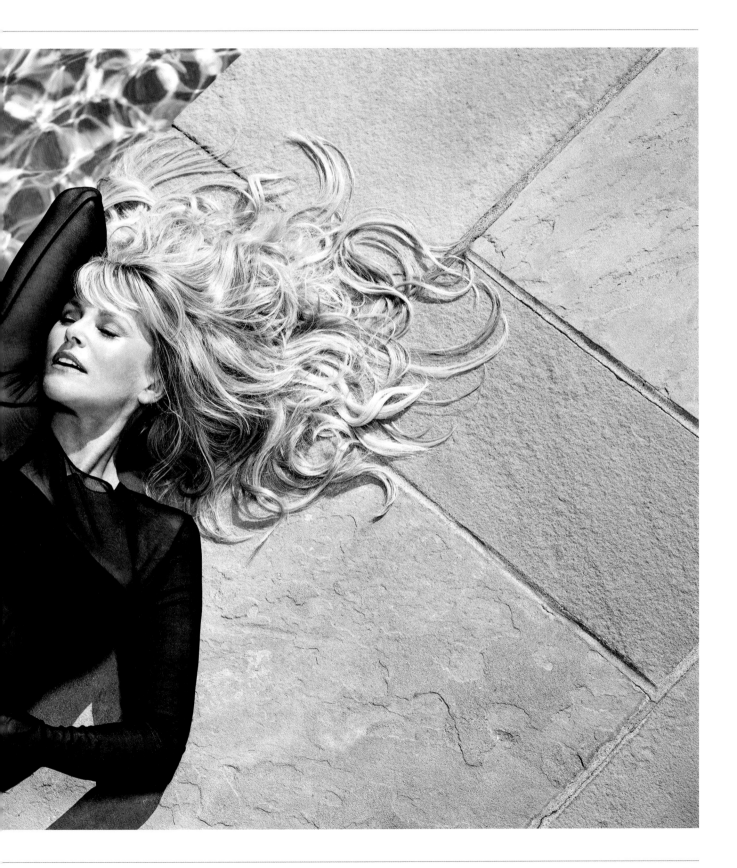

MEET THE HAIRSTYLIST:
Jen Atkin

I met Jen for the first time when she did my hair for the *Sports Illustrated Swimsuit: 50 Years of Beautiful* television special. My daughter Sailor (just starting her career as a model and very in the know) actually brought her to my attention. I had admired Jen's work in magazines, and I followed her on Instagram. So I was really excited to be able to work with her for this big event!

Not only did Jen succeed in making my hair look amazing, but she also taught me so much while I was sitting in her chair. And every time we've worked together since, I've learned even more!

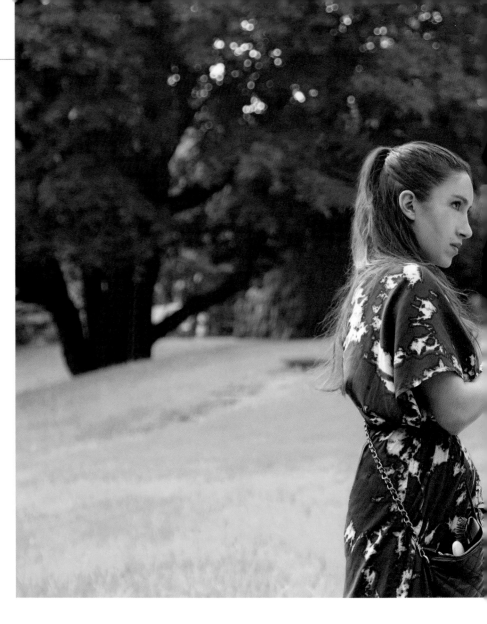

MASTER CLASS WITH JEN

"Prep your hair to hold a style or an updo by using sugar water. It's an old-fashioned trick, but it works better than any product out there. Mix a packet of white sugar into a spray bottle of water and spritz it through your hair.

"If you've got an oily scalp and dry ends (which a lot of women—especially with long hair—do), use two different sham-poos. Wash your roots with a volumiz-ing shampoo and the ends with a more moisturizing formula.

"The number one complaint I hear from women is that their hair is damaged, but no one does anything about it! Use a leave-in conditioner or an oil treatment that's right for your hair type every week. You can sleep with it in, put it in while you're taking a spin class, or during a day at the beach.

"Don't guess what products and for-mulas are best for your hair type—ask your stylist for recommendations and a professional opinion.

"To trim your own bangs, use a cuticle scissors and cut with the blades pointed up—never cut straight across."

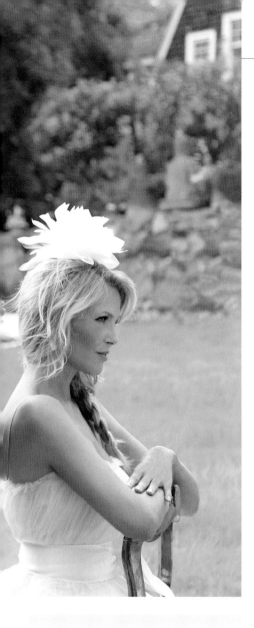

MAXIMIZE YOUR TIME WITH SOME MULTI-TASKERCISE!

When I'm drying my hair, there's not much else I can do (too noisy to talk on the phone, my hands are occupied so I can't make lists or write notes). But that's why it's the perfect time to do some of my favorite multitasking exercises. A couple of sets of squats or a few chair sits (where you squat down like you're sitting in a chair and hold there for 30 seconds or so) are easy to pull off while you're drying and styling (see pages 76–77 and 128 for more ideas on multi-taskercising).

PRODUCT RAVE

Oribe Dry Texturizing Spray is the perfect mix between a hair spray and a dry shampoo that really adds fullness and texture. I always use it before I put my hair in a ponytail because it helps hold the hair band in place in my fine, slippery hair. Some powdered sprays can make hair feel heavy and take away the shine, but not this one! (A similar product that I also love is **Philip B Russian Amber Imperial Insta-Thick Hair Thickening & Finishing Spray**— it's a body-building mist that adds oomph to fine hair.)

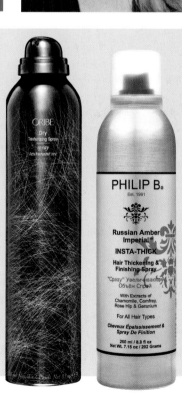

QUICK TIP
SAVE TIME DRYING

Before you reach for the blow-dryer, soak up as much excess water as you can with a super-absorbent microfiber towel (I like the ones by **Aquis**). When strands are about 80 percent dry, you can grab your dryer and brushes and start styling. The whole process will be faster and easier.

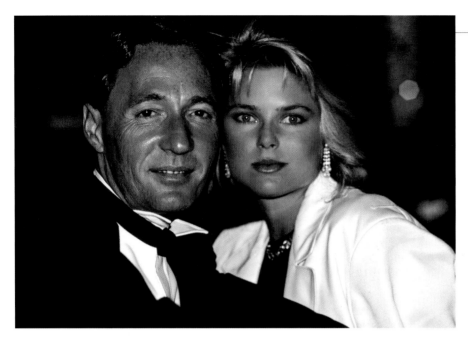

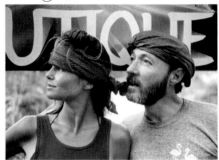

Hops and I go way back. Our adventures would make a great book!

MEET THE HAIRSTYLIST:
Maury Hopson

"I have been working with Christie since the seventies. I don't remember the exact moment we met, but I do remember that we were just instantly friends. She has such a remarkable personality and sense of humor—always full of fun! And of course, she just has such wonderful hair, which is such a pleasure for me to work with and makes my job so much easier."

MASTER CLASS WITH MAURY

"Always use a wide-toothed comb to untangle wet hair—never a hairbrush! And don't just yank and pull at your temples. Start in the back and gently work your way around toward your face. You'll lose a lot less hair that way.

"Don't throw away the nozzle attachment that comes with the blow-dryer—it's there for a reason. The nozzle directs the hot air down the hair shaft so that you get more smoothness. Without it, that big opening allows air to blow in all different directions and that makes little split ends stand up and be more noticeable.

"I love the **Ceramicare** round brushes for styling. They have uniform rows of openings that allow the warm air from your dryer to go through the brush to reach the hair. It greatly reduces the amount of time spent blow-drying.

"It's okay to hang on to a style for years—so long as you update it regularly. Adding some layers around the face or making it a little shorter can give it a more modern look.

"Don't go more than six to eight weeks between haircuts. Getting regular trims keeps your hair looking sharp, healthy, and well maintained.

"A picture is the best way to communicate with your stylist. Clients don't typically speak 'hair,' so the terms the stylist is using might not mean the same thing to them. But a picture can help your stylist more easily interpret what you're talking about and make sure you're both on the same page."

MEET THE HAIRSTYLIST:
Mitch Barry

Mitch and I have done so many jobs together over the years. He's always a joy to work with and he always works wonders with my hair! Our craziest job ever was when I had to be on TV shows on both coasts on the same day. I started the day with morning shows on the East Coast and ended the day as a presenter at a music awards show in Los Angeles. It was quite a marathon, but Mitch was more than up to the challenge. Plus we laughed and had fun the entire trip.

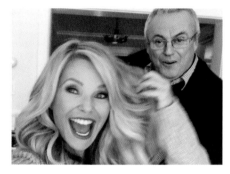

MASTER CLASS WITH MITCH

"I first worked with Christie in 1988 on a shoot for *Self* magazine. She was then, and still is, amazing to work with. She's so inspiring and we always have such a good time. But my favorite times of working with Christie were when I did her hair for *Chicago the Musical*. I had the most fun because she was having the time of her life. It was such a dream come true for her, and she really took on that character fully every single night."

"I have a lot of favorite products, but there's one I use on nearly every client. That's **Sally Hershberger Plump Up Collagen Thickening Mist**. I've never met a woman who didn't want more volume and body, and this really does the job. Spray it on your roots and then blow-dry.

"One hairbrush can't do everything. Just like you wouldn't have just one makeup brush and expect to use it to apply all your makeup, using just one hairbrush won't accomplish everything your hair needs. At the very least, I'd recommend having one that's safe to use on wet hair, a round brush for styling, and a paddle brush for smoothing dry hair.

"It's important that your stylist understand your overall style, so when you get your hair cut, dress as you want to look. If you want a polished style, don't show up in your workout clothes. If you want something easy and casual, don't arrive in a business suit.

"It seems obvious that you need to treat your hair with respect, but the biggest mistake I see women making is overprocessing their hair and overusing heat-styling tools, both of which will damage your hair.

"Hair needs rest days. It's going to be happier and healthier if you give it a day off from shampooing and styling every other day. It gives hair a break and gives the natural oils in the scalp a chance to do their work.

"When you do shampoo, focus on cleaning the roots. You don't need to scrub the ends because it'll leave them dried out and damaged.

"Long hair is youthful (just look at Christie!). And the old rules no longer apply that you can't have long hair as you get older. If you feel great with it, do it."

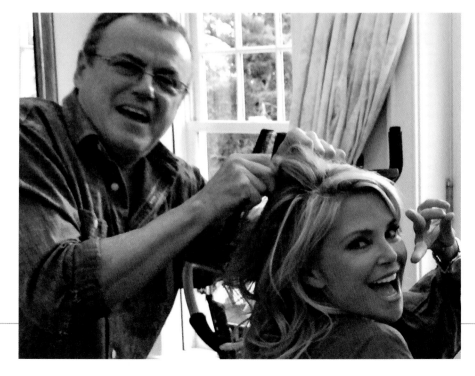

MEET THE HAIR COLORIST: *Sharon Dorram*

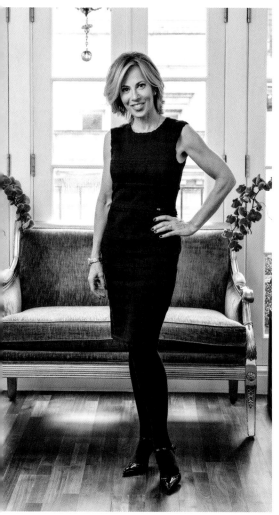

I've been trusting my color to Sharon for over ten years. When I first went to see her, my hair was overhighlighted, making it look just like a solid mass of blond. She is an artist in the way she works with color, and she helped take my hair to a new, much more flattering shade. By adding some darker color to it, she created the contrast necessary to make my blond come to life. And what I really love is that when I'm sitting in her chair, I learn so much: about hair, sure, but that's just the beginning. Sharon always knows the latest in everything from nutrition to how to get a good night's sleep (her secret is melatonin). My hair becomes golden, and it's a golden opportunity to learn something new too!

MASTER CLASS WITH SHARON

"Don't stray too far from the natural color that your hair is now. Staying within a shade or two will be more flattering to your face and your skin tone.

"Use single-process color to cover gray only as a last resort. I like to work with the gray rather than trying to completely cover it up, by adding highlights and lowlights that are closest to your real hair color. It will grow out more naturally, which means easier maintenance and less obvious roots.

"New to hair color? Err on the side of less. You can always add more, but too many highlights or too severe a color will wash out your skin tone—and you'll have to wait months for it to completely grow out.

"If you get bad hair color from someone, don't get back in their chair! Chances are, they won't know how to fix it and you'll end up damaging your hair with repeated treatments. Either live with it until it grows out, or find someone else who really can fix the problem.

"For really obvious roots, take a little bit of eye shadow in a shade that matches your hair and dab it on near your part. Anything temporary like that, that washes right out, will work in a pinch.

"Stay away from styling products that contain alcohol. It dries out the hair, which is especially harmful to hair that's been color treated.

"My own hair is really fine, so when I need to give it a boost, I use **Sally Hershberger Supreme Lift Root Spray**. It instantly amplifies your hair's volume."

ANTIAGING SECRET
GET THE RIGHT COLOR

"The biggest mistake I see women make with their hair color is having it be too one-dimensional," says Dorram. "When your color is all one shade, it lacks depth, which makes you look older. Seeing a deeper base color (no matter if you're blond, brunette, or redhead) beneath the highlights is youthful."

My hair care tool kit

I love trying new products—especially when one of my trusted experts recommends them—and there are a few that have become my tried-and-tested favorites. Here are some I can't live without:

IONIC HAIR DRYER

I think the science behind ionic dryers is intriguing, and if there's a chance it'll make my hair shinier, it's worth a try! They're available in all price ranges—**Pantene** and **Revlon** have moderately priced versions, and I see lots of hairdressers using the **Solano Supersolano 3300 xtralite** hair dryer (which I also love because it comes in chic white).

CURLING IRONS

I have two—one with a large barrel to create loose curls, and one with a smaller barrel for tighter, longer-lasting curls. I also love the shine it adds to my hair as it smooths down the hair cuticle. Look for one that has temperature settings (not just "high" and "low")—that gives you more control over the level of heat you're using.

ORIBE GRANDIOSE HAIR PLUMPING MOUSSE

It makes my hair look twice as thick. Sometimes, I'll use this together with **Oribe Maximista Thickening Spray** to create even more volume! (It's also the perfect thing to spray where I'm going to snap on an extension to add grip and hold.)

SUN-IN

Yes, I still use the same stuff we were spritzing on our hair in the '70s! It's a great way to add a few very natural-looking highlights to blond hair, and helps me extend the time between salon visits. Spray it on a cotton ball and rub it just on the strands you want to lighten.

TERAX LIFE DROPS

I rub a little of this leave-in conditioner on my ends because it really helps to get rid of the frayed look of split ends.

PRELL SHAMPOO

I used to represent Prell many years ago, and I still reach for it on occasion when I want my hair to be at its cleanest and fluffiest. Anything that's deposited in your hair—styling products, oils, hard minerals from the water—use Prell, and boom, it's out.

L'ORÉAL PARIS ELNETT SATIN HAIRSPRAY EXTRA STRONG HOLD (UNSCENTED)

This is the classic hair spray you'll find in almost every hairdresser's kit. It never makes hair feel sticky or gooey. It holds, even after you brush your hair and restyle it. I also spray it on my hairbrush at the first sign of static electricity to remove the static.

RITA HAZAN ROOT CONCEALER

If gray or dark roots start to show before you have time to get to your colorist, just spritz this onto your part. It can also be used to make hair look thicker. Just lift the top layer and spray a darker shade on the layers underneath—the depth of color under your lighter shade creates the illusion of volume, plus the spray gives hair a thicker texture.

A WATER FILTER

People don't realize how much of an effect the water you're washing in has on the health and beauty of your hair. Hard water deposits minerals on your hair that can dull your color and make hair brittle. Water that's too soft feels almost slimy and makes it hard to thoroughly rinse shampoo out of your hair. Spending the money on a filter system for your home, or even just one that attaches to your showerhead, is so worth it!

MASON PEARSON BRUSH

I use this boar bristle brush to smooth my hair when it's dry. The natural bristles stimulate the scalp to keep hair shiny and healthy.

DENMAN BRUSH

This is a classic that I've been using for years. The rounded-end nylon bristles are gentle enough for detangling wet hair, and it's great for styling too.

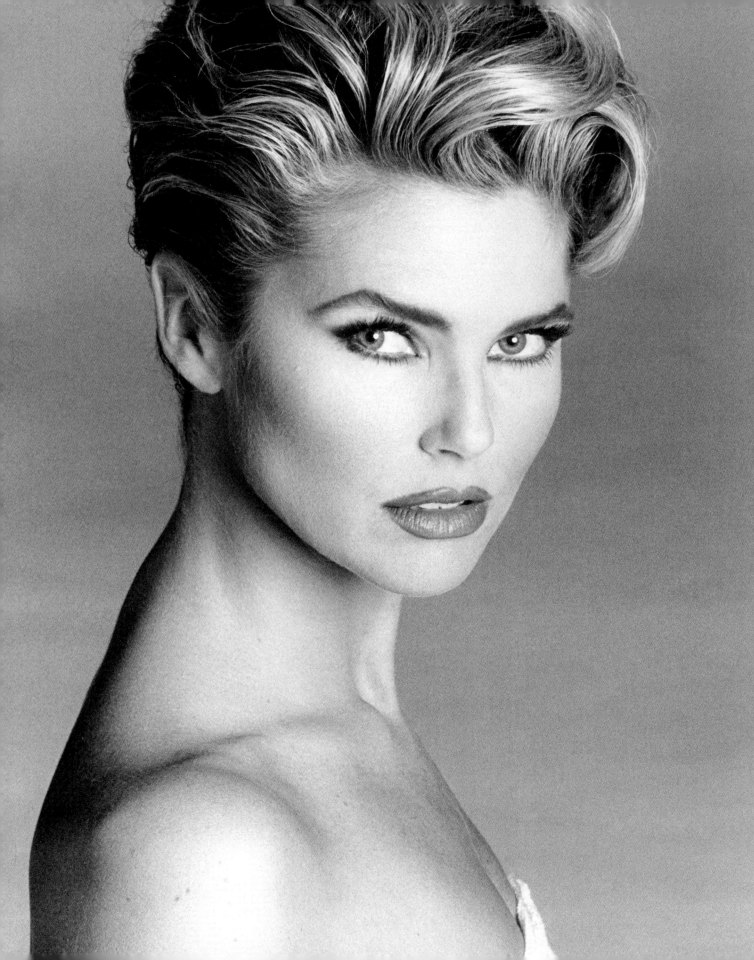

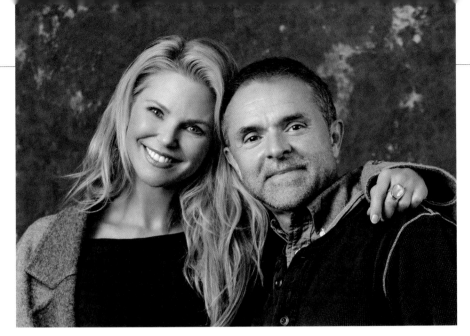

QUICK TIP
NIGHTTIME 'DO FOR LONG HAIR
I like to sleep with my hair in a top-knot. I think it helps prevent wear and tear on my hair while I sleep, plus I like the extra volume I get when I let it down in the morning.

MEET THE TRICHOLOGIST:
Kevin Mancuso

What is a trichologist, you ask? Well, I asked the same thing when Kevin—an amazing hairstylist I've worked with many, many times over the years—told me he had studied to become one. Turns out, trichology is basically the science of hair. So Kevin now not only knows everything about how to style hair, but he also knows everything about how to care for it from the inside out.

MASTER CLASS WITH KEVIN

"Beware of styling products that contain heavy silicones and oils. They will soften hair too much—making it difficult to build volume and structure. This is especially important as you get older and may have thinner hair than you used to.

"Find products that support your hair's natural texture, not fight it.

"Stress can affect the health of your hair. Going through a stressful event can leave more strands in the 'resting' phase instead of the 'growth' phase—meaning hair can look noticeably thinner. So finding ways to cope with and relieve stress will also have a positive effect on how your hair looks.

"Protein is critical for keeping hair healthy, and many people don't get enough. Lean meats, fish, eggs, and soy products are all good sources. Make sure you're getting at least one serving a day.

"During menopause, the drop in estrogen can cause an increase in male hormones—and that can lead to hair loss. Luckily, various treatments can help, including minoxidil, lasers, topical niacin, and biotin.

"You can camouflage hair loss with root-thickening products like **Super Million Hair Enhancement Fibers**. The fibers are charged with static electricity so that they bond to your existing strands and make hair look thicker.

"Hair gets increasingly susceptible to damage as you get older. To prevent breakage (which can make hair look even thinner), use a hair strengthening treatment on a regular basis. I like **Nexxus Emergencée Reconstructing Treatment**—it's got a blend of proteins, elastin, and collagen that make hair more resilient."

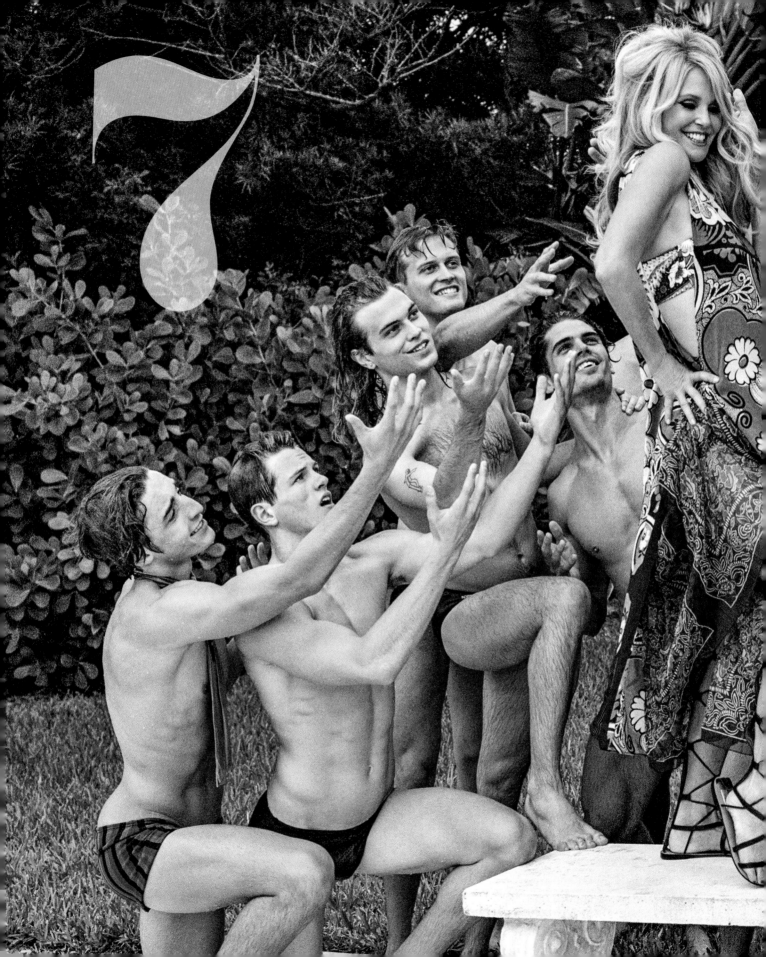

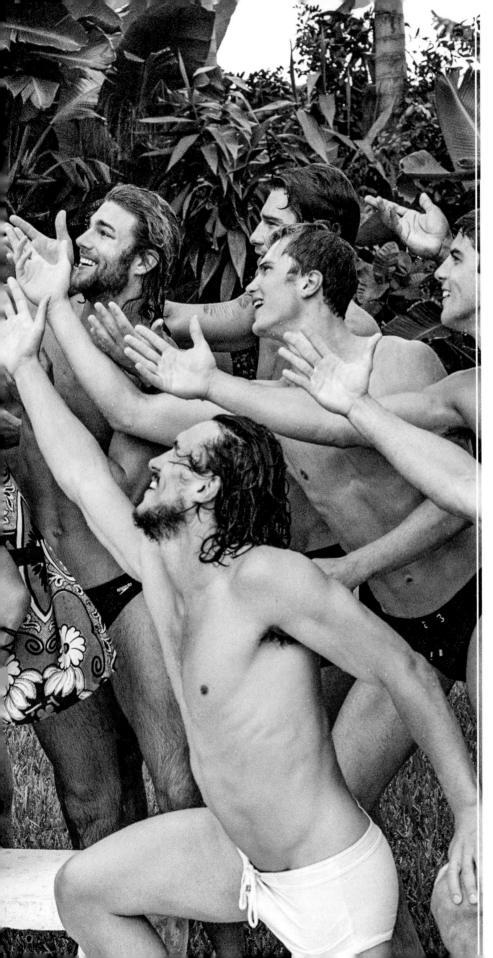

FASHION NOTEBOOK

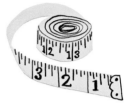

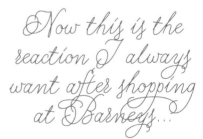

Now this is the reaction I always want after shopping at Barneys...

So which one of you is Barney, anyway?

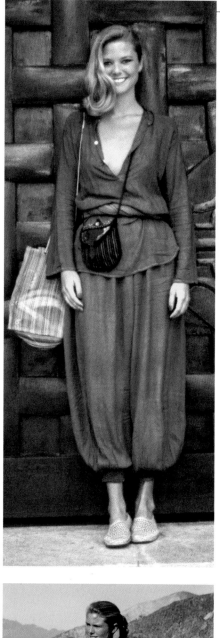

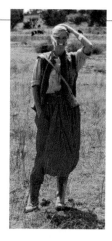

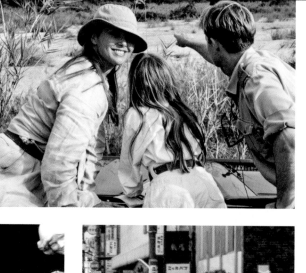

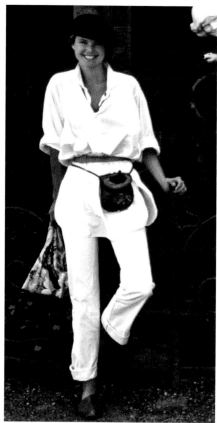

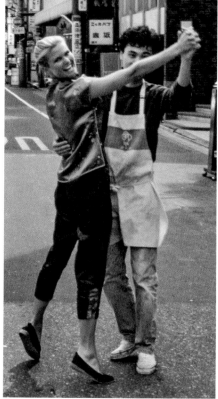

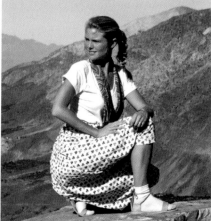

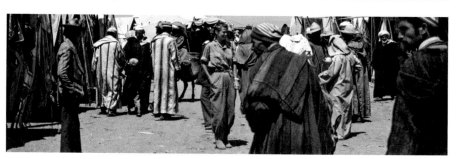

I BELIEVE

that your personal style should be about more than just clothes—it should be a reflection of who you are, where you've been, and the things you love. Thanks to my job and travels around the world, it's been easy for me to accumulate a rather eclectic closet. My kids never had to buy Halloween costumes—they just went into my closet and came out as cowgirls, American Indians, Japanese Kabuki characters, Frida Kahlo, flappers, sailors, you name it! I have clothes and accessories gathered from every corner of the world, every hobby, every adventure. I love to travel, and have always found shopping for indigenous arts and crafts, fabrics, and clothing to be a great way to get a feel for the local culture.

As you navigate the bustling medinas, *mercados*, and *grands marchés*, you get to try out your language skills, interact with the locals, and come out adorned in colorful scarves, embroidered vests, handmade sandals, straw hats, and baskets. I have djellabas from Morocco, silver bracelets and beaded necklaces from Africa, embroidered Mexican wedding dresses, huaraches, *ghos*, and turquoise from the Kingdom of Bhutan. After forty years of modeling assignments and personal adventures, I can not only come up with any Halloween

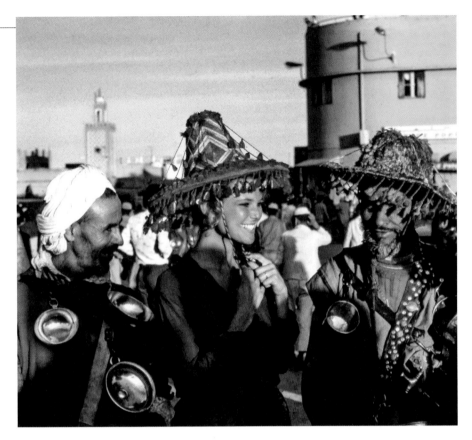

costume my kids could dream up, but I can also pull out these items to brighten up and personalize any outfit!

And if you're not the peripatetic type, there are so many online marketplaces that do the globe-trotting for you. I follow quite a few colorful sites on Instagram that offer great finds (like @gypsetgoddess and @soleil_blue). Seek out items that are unique, reflect your personality, and will add a fun flair to your wardrobe basics. But remember, whether you are shopping in a faraway place or online, NEVER buy anything made from ivory. The ivory trade has put the elephants of the world on the endangered species list and they could be extinct in as little as fifteen years, so please, SAY NO TO IVORY (more on how to get involved in this issue to come in chapter 9).

I have always loved exploring our beautiful country right here at home too. I have a passion for America's Wild West and own many Native American beaded vests and fringe jackets, vintage embroidered cowgirl and cowboy shirts, turquoise, silver bracelets, and, of course, cowboy hats, moccasins, and boots! And you don't necessarily need to be anywhere near a horse to make this Western stuff work. I just mix it all right in, the more contrasting, the better. It's more interesting and less costume-y that way. For inspiration, I look to the master of this, Ralph Lauren, and try to emulate how he mixes rugged treasures with a long skirt in a fine fabric and a jean shirt. I used to ride horses competitively, and one year I won the National Cutting Horse Association Futurity Championship in Dallas. YEE HAW! I did some two-steppin' that night! And you should have seen how I managed to work that championship buckle into every outfit for

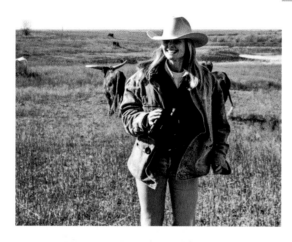

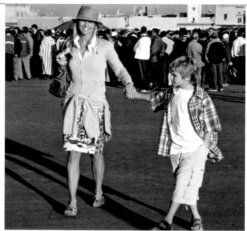

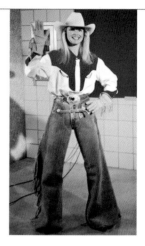

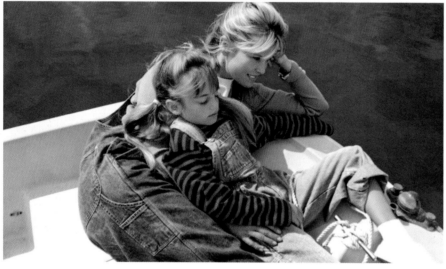

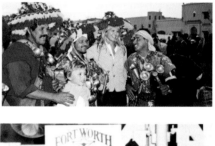

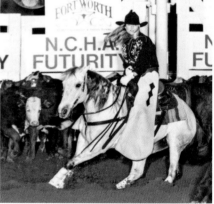

about three years straight! Talk about a conversation starter. I love having clothes and jewelry that have happy memories.

Another part of my heart, and therefore my closet, belongs to the sea. You can spot the nautical look in my closet by the piles of striped sailor shirts in every color. I also love a navy blazer—especially if there's an anchor on it! I LOVE anchors on everything from T-shirts to necklaces, and a nautical rope belt makes me feel like a castaway on a deserted island. From my beach travels, I have accumulated a great collection of pareus and sarongs, and even my jewelry box reflects my love of the sea.

My "diamonds" are seashell necklaces, bracelets, and earrings. My parents lived in Hawaii for many years, so I spent a lot of time taking dreamy walks along the beautiful Hawaiian shores, collecting puka shells and turning them into necklaces. I also make my own shell-encrusted picture frames and memory boxes for my kids to keep precious items, like their first baby bootie, rattle, and letters to the tooth fairy.

My point in sharing all this is to show you that fashion really should be fun and personal. So, think of where you've been that makes you happy and try to incorporate the feel of that place into your everyday outfits whenever

possible. Do you like the West? Then wear a jean jacket over those black pants or add some turquoise to your jewelry collection. Or if you love the mountains, add a ski sweater and some stylish warm boots to your winter wardrobe. And don't be afraid to bring back a few colorful scarves or pareus from your tropical beach vacation. Every time you wear one to the neighborhood pool or wrap it around your neck as a scarf, you'll have a vivid reminder of a wonderful trip!

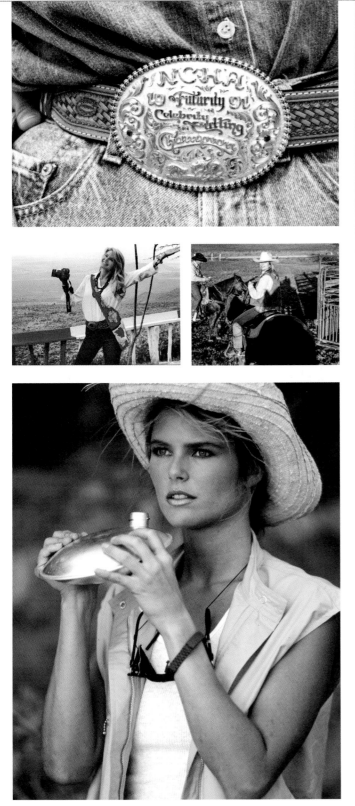

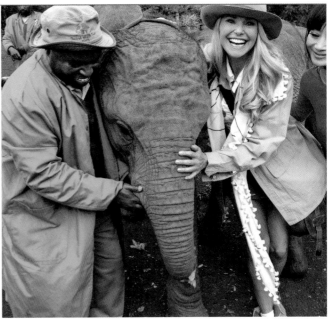

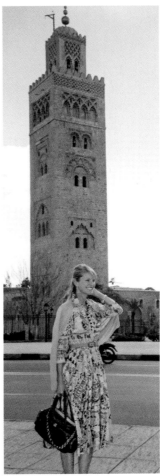

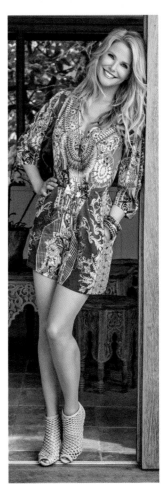

The basics every woman should own

In addition to my eclectic travel finds, I've also accumulated a wonderful wardrobe of truly classic pieces over the years. Trends come and go, but certain timeless items are always in style. Build a wardrobe of these go-to pieces (in go-with-everything colors like black, gray, white, khaki, and navy), and you'll never be left with that "I have nothing to wear" feeling. And it's worth it to spend a little more on classics that will last through the years. Then mix them up with all those fun, personal accessories you collect to truly make them your own.

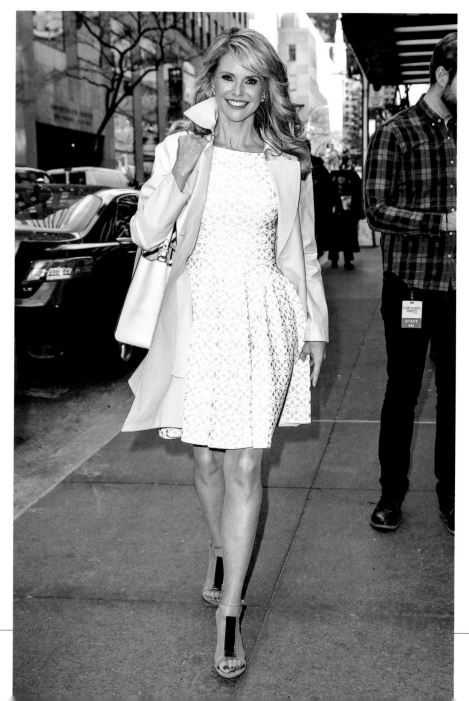

ARE THESE TIMELESS PIECES IN YOUR CLOSET?

TRENCH COAT
Always a chic option, rain or shine!

PEA COAT
Another of my nautical necessities—a short pea coat is a great jacket to throw on for around town.

THE PERFECT WHITE T-SHIRT
White helps to brighten up your face. Find one that fits your body perfectly—it should have a little Lycra in it.

TANK TOPS
White is classic, but I also keep a couple in black, khaki, and gray and layer them under everything from T-shirts to dress shirts to blazers.

STRIPED SAILOR SHIRT
Looks as great with jeans as it does with anything else you can think of!

A CRISP WHITE DRESS SHIRT
A cotton men's-style dress shirt never goes out of style. Wear it with jeans (tucked or untucked), with dressier trousers, or a pencil skirt. And as Sharon Stone once proved at the Oscars, it really can take you anywhere.

A GREAT SIMPLE JACKET
A tailored blazer or a bomber jacket (which is an updated version of a blazer) can go from the office to your kid's soccer game.

OVERSIZED TURTLENECKS & CREW NECKS
Everyone needs a comfy sweater they can throw on with leggings, jeans, or even a slim skirt.

A PAIR OF REAL PANTS
A classic trouser that goes straight down from the widest part of your hips, with maybe a slight flare at the bottom, is a true wardrobe staple.

A SELECTION OF JEANS
Classic cuts or trendy, make sure they really fit your body. (More on these in a minute.)

A SIMPLE PENCIL SKIRT
You can pair it with your white dress shirt and jacket for instant polish.

A FULL SKIRT
One in a "fancy" fabric can be dressed up or down depending on what you pair with it.

A PAIR OF GREAT PUMPS
In whatever color you wear most (black, brown, navy). Also, having a nude pair that exactly matches your skin tone is a great way to make your legs look longer!

A PAIR OF COMFORTABLE FLATS
I always have white leather Stan Smiths, navy espadrilles, and tan leather sandals in my closet.

BOOTS
I love to wear flat, knee-high, or over-the-knee boots with skinny jeans and an oversized sweater. And a slightly refined version of a motorcycle boot updates a look.

A COOL PAIR OF SNEAKERS
I like slip-on versions, like Vans, in a fun print like leopard or camouflage.

A COUPLE OF GREAT HATS
I love fedoras, berets, Panama hats, and beanies. A hat can complete a look in a fun way. (And help rescue you on a bad hair day!)

Jeans: your wardrobe's best friend

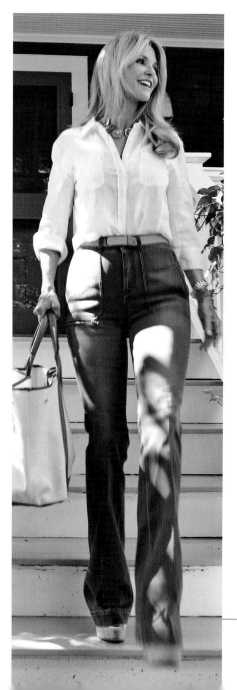

I really do live in jeans. And that's easy to do these days, because with the variety of styles and colors available, you can wear them almost anywhere. Jean styles change so fast today that I think it makes following "jean rules" kind of an obsolete notion. If a pair flatters my figure, is super comfy, or holds special memories, I keep them. That said, here are some guidelines for finding—and wearing—that perfect pair:

- Don't try to pour yourself into a too-tight pair for size bragging rights. We can't see what size you're wearing, and jeans that are too small are not only uncomfortable, but unflattering too.
- Find the right rise. The "rise" is the technical term for the distance from the seam at the crotch up to the waistband. One that's too low can leave you over-exposed (and even create a muffin top you didn't know you had!), and one that's too high just screams "mom jeans!" Look for a flattering mid-rise that keeps your butt and tummy covered but still falls several inches below your belly button.
- The color of your denim is up to your personal preference, but the most flattering, slimming choice for most women (especially those past their forties!) is a dark blue wash. I call these my "fancy jeans," because paired with a blazer or nice cashmere sweater, they work even for a casual business meeting or dinner out.

QUICK TIP
LOSE THE LOVE HANDLES
If you're getting dressed in your jeans and don't like the way your stomach looks, let that be your impetus for cranking out a set of planks (see page 70 for details on how to do them correctly). Relating your exercise directly to getting dressed will help you stay motivated. Just think how much better those jeans are going to look if you keep this up!

- My jeans collection features every style you can think of, but if you're going to invest in only a few key pairs, go for classic styles—like straight leg, boot cut, or trouser—that can be dressed up or down and worn for work or on weekends.
- Just as with the rest of your wardrobe, pulling together the perfect jeans pairing is all about proportions. Wider leg styles (boot cut, trouser) look best with chunkier heels, while skinnier, straight-leg styles go well with more delicate pumps or slim boots. I still love slouchy boyfriend jeans, but you have to be really careful what you wear them with or the look will put on pounds. I often wear them when it's warmer so that I can balance them with a strappy sandal and a top that shows some skin to make the look more feminine.
- When you get your jeans hemmed (and you'll need to, in order for them to look chic, not sloppy), make sure to ask the tailor to cut off the original hem, shorten the jeans, then reattach the original hem.

ALL DRESSED UP:
A few tricks for a beautiful night out

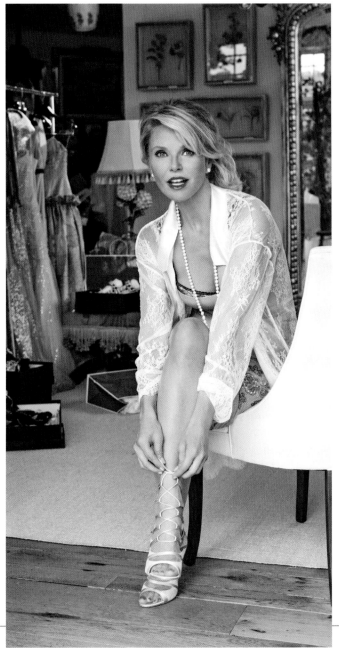

Everyone has an event now and then (whether it's a wedding, a school reunion, or just an anniversary dinner out on the town) when you really want to go for the "wow factor." When I'm getting dressed for a big event, I often go outside my comfort zone a bit. But I think the key to pulling off a successful—but still "wow"—look is to be selective in what you choose to highlight. For example, if I'm going to be daring and show some cleavage, I won't also have a skirt up to there and lots of makeup. I'm going to try to make the rest of the look very polished and ladylike. Or if I choose a very short skirt, well, I'll let my legs do the talking and make sure the rest of me is fairly covered up and modest. You get the point—highlight one feature at a time, not everything together!

An evening out is the perfect opportunity to show off a little skin and try something a bit sexier than your everyday attire. And I think every woman has some feature that's worth highlighting. The trick is to stop focusing on what's *not* working and concentrate on what is. Look for a dress that gives you a little detail somewhere that accents what you think is working. Maybe it's a long dress that's mostly covered up but with a peekaboo slit to reveal a sexy flash of leg. Or you could conceal your arms with long sleeves but have a plunging neckline that calls attention to your great cleavage. Long sleeves also work with a looser, off-the-shoulder sort of top that highlights a beautiful neck and collarbones—plus, there's always that tension of maybe it will fall down too low! If your back is in great shape, look for a style that's covered in front and open behind (or has a sheer lace inset to give the illusion of skin without actually revealing much at all). The point is, draw attention to whatever looks best, and no one will even notice that little underarm jiggle or love handle you're so worried about!

QUICK TIP
TURN YOUR CARDIGAN INTO A SHRUG
When I want a little something to cover my shoulders and upper arms, I use this trick. Put on a cardigan, pull it behind you and button the bottom button behind your back. Your cardigan is now contained behind you and looks like a shrug!

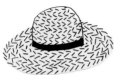

MEET THE FASHION STYLIST:
Wayne Scot Lukas

I met Wayne on a job about thirty years ago, and in a business where people often tell you whatever they think you want to hear, Wayne is very honest—sometimes even brutally so. My daughter Alexa dubbed him "the magic mirror" when she was little because when you stand in front of him, he tells you exactly what he sees!

Wayne's approach to dressing is about much more than clothes. He understands that looking good is really about confidence. You can make a paper bag look great if you wear it with an attitude that expresses and celebrates your individuality. And that's a fashion statement I will always agree with!

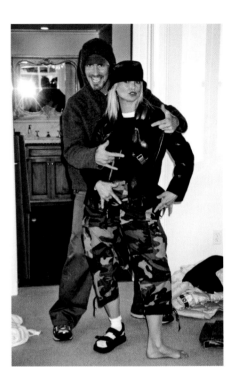

MASTER CLASS WITH WAYNE

"The biggest mistake women make is not dressing for themselves. If you spend all your time dressing to please your boyfriend, husband, boss, or friends, you're never going to learn what really works for you and makes you feel good about your body. If you only know your body as other people see it, then you don't know your body. And you can't develop a personal style when you're always dressing to please someone else.

"Take someone you love shopping—and by that I mean you! Look in the mirror before you go shopping and find something you love about your body and want to accentuate. And never go shopping when you're hungry, angry, or feeling bad about yourself.

"You can get great tips from $10,000-a-day stylists by paying attention to how they dress celebrities. If you have the same coloring or body shape as a person who regularly shows up on the pages of *People* and *Us Weekly*, then look for the colors, styles, or shapes that look good on them. You can get free advice by emulating the looks you see in those magazines.

"Each season, look for a great pair of jeans that fits, flatters, and is on trend. The right jeans can make an older top or jacket look hip again. And a good jean can be your go-to uniform—dress them up or down, you can wear jeans anywhere. When you find a pair you love, if you can afford it, buy more than

one color (black, dark blue, faded, white), and they can be the foundation of your wardrobe.

"Take compliments to heart. If several people tell you that you look great in blue, then you should buy more blue. If you get a lot of compliments on a certain style of jeans or a jacket or a dress, buy more pieces like that. It's not brain surgery!

"Get pieces of a trend; don't become the trend. If the trend is silver, don't walk down the street looking like a baked potato wrapped in tinfoil. Get a silver belt or a silver bag."

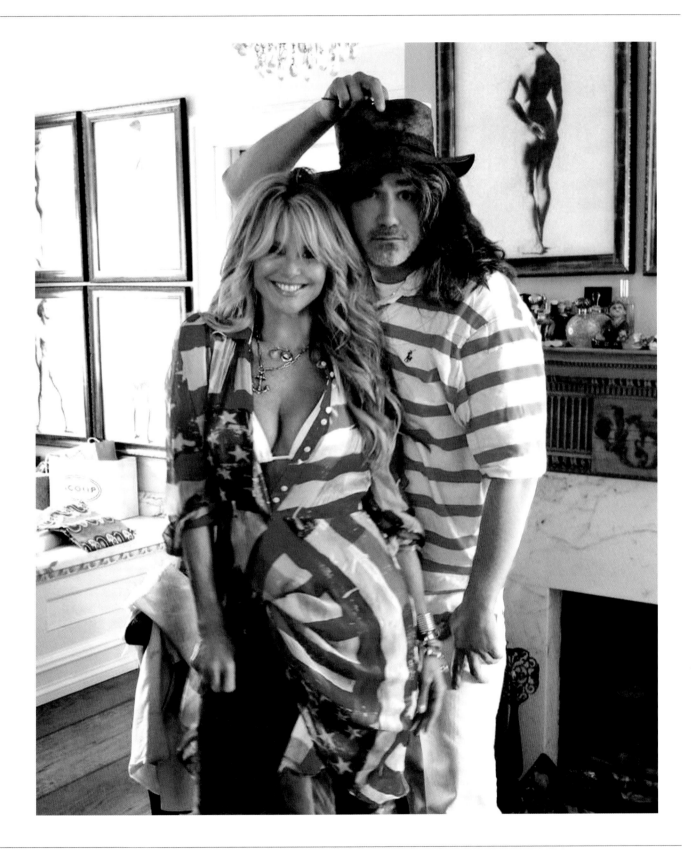

Wayne and Christie's 5 rules for dressing slimmer

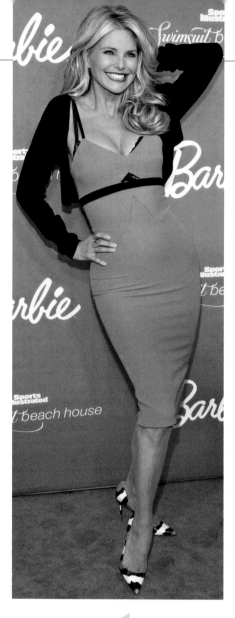

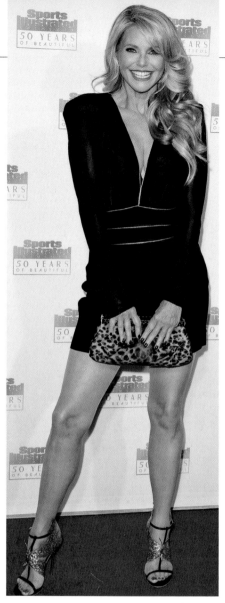

WL: Dress in clothes that fit you perfectly. Have hems taken up, a waist nipped in, or a sleeve shortened. Well-tailored clothes will always look polished and expensive (no matter how much they cost). And if you're trying to hide a bit of jiggle, more fitted clothing actually looks better than blousy, messy styles.

CB: I agree! Remember to buy clothes that fit comfortably—some buy smaller sizes for bragging rights, but comfort never goes out of style!

WL: Adding a slight shoulder pad to a shirt, dress, or jacket can help balance your look and make your hips look smaller.

CB: It's the same idea as my theory: "Big hair = smaller hips!" I feel the same way about shoes: if my shoes make my feet look too tiny, I instantly look five pounds heavier!

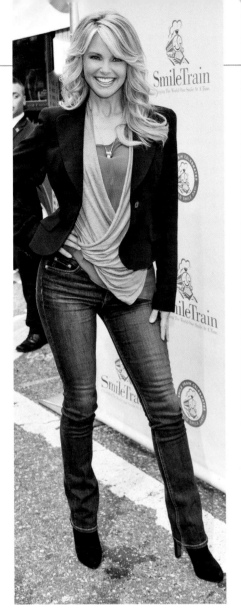

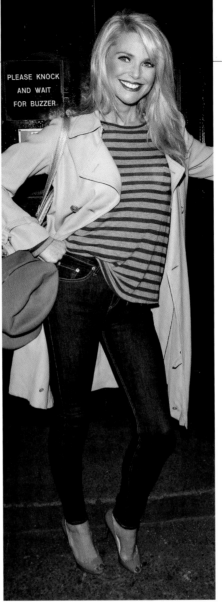

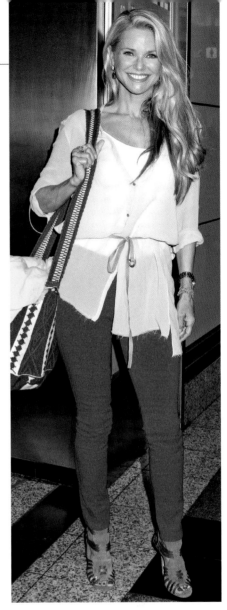

WL: A stovepipe jean that flows from the widest part of your hips straight to the floor will create a streamlined, slim look.

CB: I think the secret to looking great in jeans is the right shoe and the right rise—higher is usually better in both categories! With espadrilles and sneakers being the exception.

WL: A skinny jean with a tight ankle looks best with a structured shoe, or tuck your skinny jeans into a knee-high boot to help balance your look.

CB: I like the flexibility of a skinny jean. I can pair them with a flat, or they look sexy with over-the-knee boots in suede (which is softer looking than leather).

WL: Don't accentuate one body part at the expense of others. For example, if you're large on top but have thin legs, don't wear a huge tunic and leggings. Better to balance your top and bottom so that the overall look is slim and streamlined.

What's underneath it all

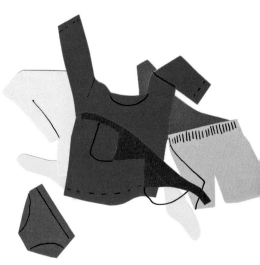

Your underwear shouldn't be an afterthought, because it really can make or break an outfit. You will look thinner and your clothes will fit better when you have on the right underpinnings. Shapewear is all the rage these days, and even though I'm not a huge fan, there are times when I rely on it. But you need to be careful which shapers you choose. They are designed to compress the body, and I find that they often create a bulge where they end. So if I do turn to a shaper, I make sure to get one that's thin (so that it doesn't actually add more bulk while trying to pull you in) and that has a flat seam rather than a sewn hem that can create a bulge. The **Commando Classic Thong** doesn't show under anything and is great when all you want is a little help holding your tummy in. And the **Trust Your Thinstincts** line from **Spanx** is so very, very lightweight and thin that they're slimming without being uncomfortable.

Probably the best thing you can do for your wardrobe is to get yourself a couple of great, perfect-fitting bras. Wearing the wrong size can wreck your look—a too-tight band will dig into your back and make bulges, and if the cups are too small you'll literally runneth over. So it pays to get measured and fitted by a professional every couple of years. Once you know your size, shop for the perfect T-shirt bra (like the **OnGossamer Sheer Bliss T-Shirt Bra**). Bring your tightest white T-shirt with you and slip it on over every bra you try on. The right one will not show at all—no ripples, no bulges, no spillage. Save the fancy, lacy bra for wearing with other things (it'll look incredibly sexy peeking out from your classic menswear shirt, for example). When you want to give your cleavage a natural-looking boost, try the **Gossard Superboost Plunge Bra.** I also love convertible bras (I'll often bring one on a job when I don't know what clothes they'll put me in). I have one by **Wacoal,** the **Red Carpet Strapless,** that's totally smooth and seamless and converts from strapless to halter, crisscross, or even one-shoulder. When I just need a reliable strapless bra that won't let me down, I reach for **Le Mystère Sculptural Strapless Bra**—it's very smooth so it doesn't show under anything but it provides nice support and coverage.

And on the bottom, well, look for something that fits your bottom! The reason some underpants give the dreaded visible panty line is that they don't fit perfectly. The right pair should lie completely smooth under your clothes—no dents or lines or bulges. **OnGossamer** makes a **mesh hip bikini** and a **mesh high-cut brief** that have soft lace edges that lie smooth against the body and never show. And **Hanky Panky thongs** have a nice wide band that lies flat around your hips.

PRODUCT RAVE

I love ultrasheer stockings by **Fogal** and **Wolford**—they are a splurge, but I think they're worth it. If you get ones that are denier 7 or lower, they are virtually invisible but make your legs look flawless. I reach for a pair of ultrasheer stockings in a shade that matches my skin as closely as possible whenever I want to wear a short skirt. It gives me more confidence—and I bet if you tried them, you'd feel like you could rock a shorter skirt too!

QUICK TIP
LOSE THE LABELS

I cut all the labels out of my underwear and slips because I don't want any extra bulges or lines showing through my clothing.

MEET THE FASHION STYLIST:
Phillip Bloch

I've worked with Phillip on and off for over twenty years, and he's helped me get dressed for some fabulous occasions—one of my favorites was a gala performance at the Metropolitan Opera in New York City. I loved the amazing black dress he found for me that was strapless and formfitting, but flared out with a few ruffles and feathers at the bottom. He paired it with a dramatic, statement-making necklace, opera-length gloves (of course!), and a scarlet clutch for a dash of color. So glamorous!

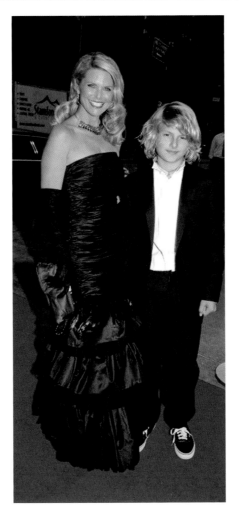

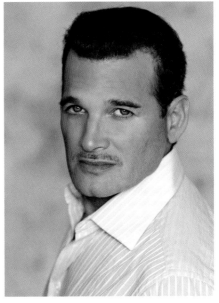

MASTER CLASS WITH PHILLIP

"If you're getting dressed and suddenly don't like what you see, don't buy into the panic. Get clinical instead and break it down piece by piece. Look at the neckline. Does that work for you? Look at the waist. Does it fit and flatter you? What about the length? The fabric? The color? Look at it intellectually rather than emotionally.

"Focus on the positive when you're getting dressed. If you love your cleavage, start by selecting a neckline that flatters it.

"If you find aspects of an outfit that you don't like, work on coming up with practical solutions. For example, if you don't like how your arms look, maybe you'd feel better if you put a cardigan over the dress.

"The biggest mistake I see women making is wearing clothes that don't fit well. Even if you only spend fifty dollars on the dress, spend another fifty dollars to get it tailored to perfection.

"Wear clothes that you are comfortable in. You'll never look great when you're fidgeting with your clothes and looking uncomfortable.

"I'm a big fan of being prepared. Have a few go-to outfits and items in your closet that you know will always work— ones you can throw on and look like a million bucks.

"Sure, you need a great dress, but the real key is your attitude. The right attitude and confidence can make any outfit look rich and expensive.

"Get your beauty sleep. Nothing makes you look better than a little rest!"

Do you need to dress your age?

You hear the phrase "age-appropriate" all the time—often in reference to clothing. For some reason, women have gotten the message that certain stylish items are off-limits after a certain age. That somewhere around middle age, you're supposed to trade in all your fashionable, chic, youthful pieces for a wardrobe of dowdy skirts and mom jeans. I turned sixty last February 2 (Groundhog Day—so does that mean I just get to keep turning sixty over and over and over?!), and I have no intention of giving up any of my favorite styles anytime soon. Certain items have been staples in my wardrobe pretty much my entire life—and I intend to keep wearing them.

I do think, though, that it's really important to dress the body you have—regardless of how old you are. So let's stop saying "age-appropriate" and start thinking about what's "body-appropriate." That's partly related to age (I know I don't have the same body I did at twenty-two), but also just about being honest with yourself. Like when I've gained a few pounds, I'm not going to reach for my skinniest jeans. Or when my shoulder injury prevented me from lifting weights for a while, I steered clear of anything sleeveless. Even if you don't feel comfortable baring your entire arm, revealing some shoulder or the part from elbow to wrist by wearing a three-quarter sleeve will look great. Wayne's always pushing my long sleeves up to show off that delicate part of the arm—and it does look younger and fresher than being all covered up.

Self tanner is another fantastic way to help you feel more comfortable revealing some skin. Slightly tanned legs look thinner, and self tanner can help camouflage any little veins or dark spots you're worried about. MAC makes a great body makeup that every makeup artist carries, **MAC Studio Face and Body Foundation**—it's great for your arms, legs, chest, and it doesn't stain your clothes. (In case you missed it, I talk about all my favorite tanning products in chapter 4.)

But no matter what age you are or whether or not your body is looking exactly as you'd like it to, staying true to yourself and your own personal style is always going to make you look and feel your best!

QUICK TIP

WEAR A BATHING SUIT WITH CONFIDENCE

I made my living in bathing suits for many, many years—and even at sixty I still dare to wear a bikini now and then. I think the key to a flattering bathing suit is in the structure. Look for suits with underpinnings that support your chest and keep your tummy and rear looking tight. I also like one-pieces or tankinis that have ruching on the sides—it's very forgiving if you want to be able to sit up and not have people count how many places your stomach folds over! And don't forget about your cover-up—a sarong, caftan, or long skirt is not only great for wearing to and from the beach or pool, but also for protecting your skin from the sun!

TIMELESS vs. DATED

Being aware of trends and staying current makes you look effortlessly stylish.	Too many trends at once will make you look silly (not chic!).
Soft fabrics—like cashmere, soft cotton, and silk—subliminally say "young, soft skin."	Stiff, wrinkly, pleated fabrics can emphasize wrinkles on your skin.
Showing a little skin.	Showing too much or covering up too much.

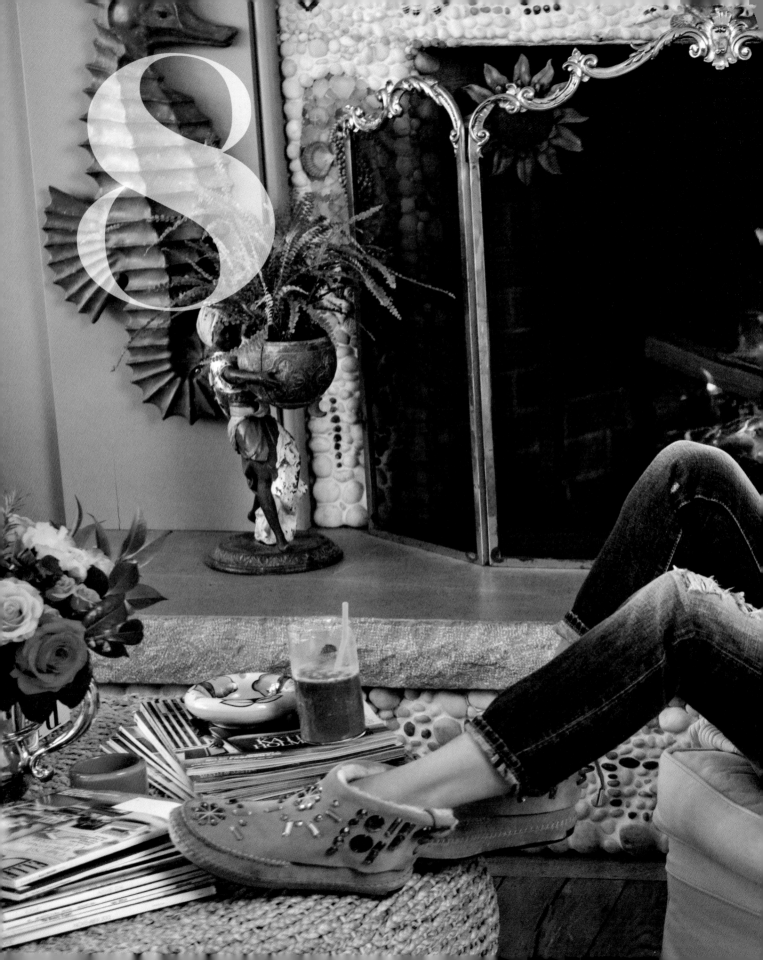

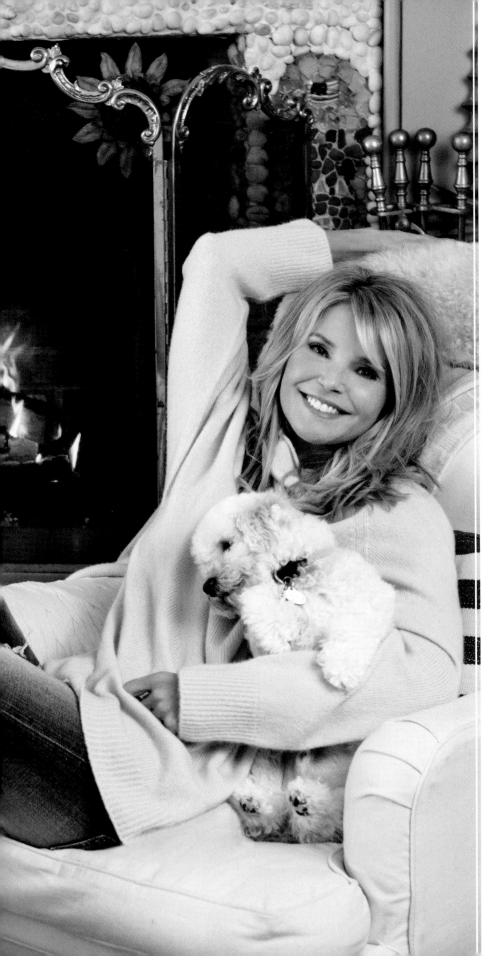

YOU ASKED, I ANSWERED

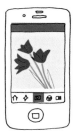

Being curious about the world around you is a beautiful trait that keeps you young at heart!

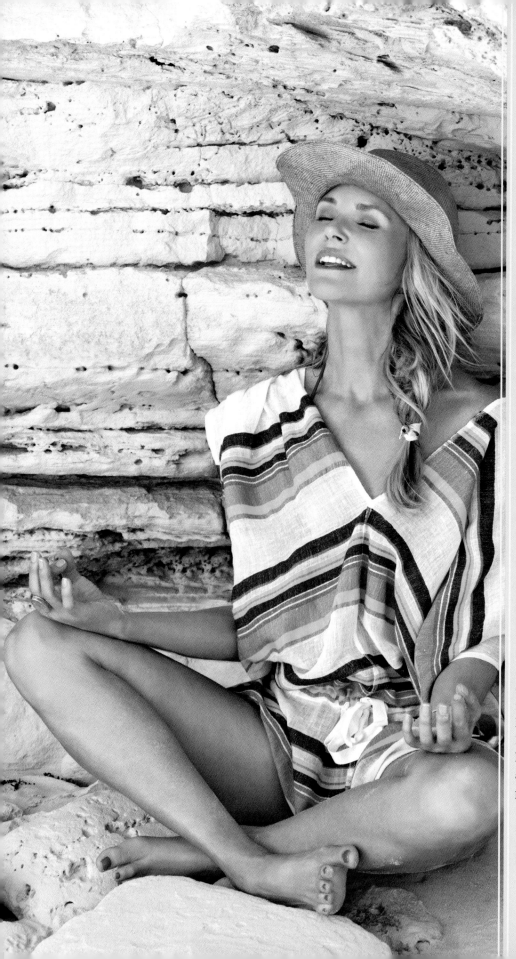

WHEN

you want to get a consensus, opinions, an idea of what people are thinking, where do you turn? You guessed correctly...Social media! There's no shortage of opinions out there, sometimes more than you want (ouch!). But in the social media lottery, I definitely lucked out. Somehow, my accounts are full of really cool, kind, fun, interesting (and interested), accomplished people from every walk of life, many countries, and diverse occupations and passions. I have often been touched and impressed by the kindness, compassion, knowledge, and thoughtfulness of the comments and posts on my pages. So when I decided I needed a little help with this book, naturally I turned to my friends on Facebook and Instagram. And they did not let me down! Many of the questions you suggested were about things I have included in other chapters, so thank you—that helped me know I was on the right track. But here are a few great questions that I hadn't thought of. See, I told you I have a lot of smart, thoughtful people on my pages. Thank you!

@christiebrinkley

What is your favorite go-to item of clothing?

I love jeans! I know that's not unique, but I don't think anything is as versatile or as practical as a pair of jeans. I can dress them up or dress them down. They never wrinkle. They're great for traveling. I have jeans in every style—distressed, ripped, torn, faded, dark, shiny, baggy, skinny, sailor, painter, flared, bells, boot cut, high-waisted, cropped, you name it! And if you missed it, in chapter 7 I share some tips for buying and wearing them.

Do you count calories?

I have counted enough calories in my lifetime to know that I don't want to count any more calories! And I don't have to—and you don't either. Because once you stop "deny-iting" (you know, dieting so all you can think of is the food you think you're denying yourself), and start focusing on eating healthy, delicious foods, you won't have to worry about calories. The foods you reach for will contain healthy oils—not artery-clogging fats—essential vitamins, and other nutrients; and the calories you consume in your healthy choices will easily be converted into the fuel you need to power you through your day. So you must have an awareness of what you're eating, and opt for fresh, unprocessed foods whenever possible. When you eat food that comes with a label (in other words, anything in a package), you do need to read what's in it and even how many calories it has. But things like fresh fruits and vegetables, lean meats, fish, and whole grains are never going to add up to the kind of calories you need to worry about. Just eat them (in reasonable portion sizes, of course) and enjoy all the nutritional goodness they deliver! I give you much more information about a healthy diet to chew on in chapter 2.

> **QUICK TIP**
> ## YOUR JEANS DON'T LIE
> While I don't count calories (or even get on the scale very often), I do have a pair of what I like to call my "honest jeans." They're the pair that fits me perfectly when I'm at my ideal weight. So if I'm ever worried that I may have put on a few pounds, I slip into those (or try to!) and they never lie to me.

How can I make my hair look shinier?

There are many ways to add shine to your hair, but one of them can also be the culprit in what causes the damage that dulls hair—and that's heat. A hair dryer with a styling brush or a flat iron can work wonders to smooth the hair cuticle and increase shine. But before you reach for any heated styling tools, reach for a product that protects and actually uses the heat to repair and condition your hair. I like to add **Kérastase Resistance Ciment Thermique** to my ends before I blow-dry (it's a heat-activated reconstructing milk that protects hair). When my hair has been overworked and overprocessed, I apply that and then tame my broken flyaways with a medium-barrel curling iron because the heat adds so much shine.

There are also products that coat your hair to give it shine. These tend to contain slippery silicone, which I personally find weighs my hair down. But there are a few shine-enhancers I've found that are lightweight but still work (like **Terax Life Drops** and **Oribe Gel Sérum Radiance, Magic and Hold**).

And don't overlook your kitchen! What you eat will directly impact your hair (plus, some foods make great DIY hair treatments). Take avocados, for example—eat half to get the healthy mono- and poly-unsaturated fats it contains, then smash up the other half and use it as a hair mask. Wash it out and you'll see how your hair shines! See chapter 6 for more tips on how food affects your hair health.

QUICK TIP
COCONUT KEEPS HAIR SLEEK

If you have long hair, you can use a small amount of coconut oil on the ends to make them look sleek and shiny. Just don't slather it all over your hair and scalp—it's very nourishing, but you'll do more damage trying to shampoo it out! I occasionally put it on the lower half of my hair and then rub the excess from my hands on the top half for an hour before shampooing.

How can I apply eye makeup to make my eyes appear bigger?

Making your eyes look bigger is all about where you place the shadow, and we really get into the details in chapter 5 (with loads of info directly from some of the top makeup artists in the business). But when I'm in a hurry, I use a brown pencil to fill in the spaces along my lash line and that, plus curling my lashes and putting on a quick coat of mascara, completely wakes up my eyes. I'll also take my blush and do a quick sweep over my eyelids. If you've got more time, extend the liner a little farther at the outer edge of your eye and soften it with a smudge of eye shadow. Adding a few clumps of false lashes on the outer corner of the upper lash line can really emphasize the eyes and make them look dramatically larger (in chapter 5 you'll also find how-tos for applying those falsies).

How do you make thinning eyebrows look lush?

Again, take a look at chapter 5 for some great tips on shaping and enhancing your eyebrows. You would be surprised how strengthening a brow can add dimension and uplift to your face, and literally take years off!

To give you a quick answer to your question, I like to use a brow pencil in a light taupe or medium to dark blond to make light, feathery strokes in the direction that your brows naturally grow. You can soften it—and add even more dimension to your brows—by going over it with a brow brush dipped into an eye shadow that matches your brow color. **Giorgio Armani Eye & Brow Maestro** is a kit that does it all—use it to fill in your eyelash line, your brows, and even cover thin spots in your hairline or your gray roots! Use a slanted brow brush with fairly hard bristles so you can really get in between the hairs to shade and add fullness. When I'm in a rush, I just use powder because it's most natural looking and forgiving.

What supplements do you take on a regular basis?

Here's a list of my daily vitamins and supplements:

BIOSIL (FOR MY HAIR, SKIN, AND NAILS)

CURCUMIN C3 COMPLEX 500 MG

ESTER-C 500 MG

ACETYL L-CARNITINE 250 MG

COENZYME Q10 100 MG

B6 COMPLEX

L-ARGININE 500 MG

VITAMIN D3 2000 IU

CALCIUM

FOLIC ACID 800 MG

MULTI B VITAMIN

After my warm lemon water first thing in the morning, I have a **Bio-K** yogurt because I believe probiotics keep me healthy! You can get them in both dairy and dairy-free versions, and I think they are the best probiotics. There are also probiotic drinks like kombucha and **KeVita**, which are really delicious—just watch out for the sugar content.

Now, it's really important for me to note that these are the supplements I've decided work for *me*. But everyone's needs are different, so please don't take my list as any sort of gospel! I firmly believe that you should do your own research, and talk to a nutritionist and to your doctor in order to come up with a personalized prescription that suits you best. Also, I tend to mix it up occasionally, switching formulas and vitamins—just as I do with my diet and exercise—so I don't get stuck in a rut.

What is the very first thing you do every morning?

I throw open my curtains and say, "THANK YOU!" Then I make my cup of warm water with lemon. Sometimes I add a little honey to the top edge of the cup and dip it in cayenne powder or cinnamon—the combination helps cleanse and flush out toxins, and it contains vitamin C to boost the immune system and potassium to feed brain and nerve cells. It's a great way to start the day!

What are your thoughts on Botox, fillers, face-lifts, etc.?

Let's start with face-lifts. I don't think that I, or any celebrity, should play a role in a decision that can impact your life for better or worse forever. YOU have to make that decision for yourself, along with consultation with your doctors. It's a huge life- (and face-) altering decision that can make you look as young as you feel, but it also carries risks that are best discussed with a well-researched plastic surgeon.

Now let's talk about easier, less scary choices for making your face look more youthful—and they run the gamut. There are so many new low-risk, temporary fixes, from Botox and fillers to devices that use light and sound waves to stimulate your body's own natural collagen. And I don't think there should be any shame or stigma attached to any of the above choices. But I also don't think anyone should feel pressured to try cosmetic treatments—or to think of aging or wrinkles as an affliction! It's really important to age gracefully, and to me that means being happy and comfortable in your own skin. Sometimes the most beautiful things about someone's face are the smile lines and other lines that are the souvenirs of a life of good humor and adventure. If that's the case for you, then you should happily embrace them! But if your reflection doesn't look as full of life and energy as you feel, there are lots of things you can do about it. Have a look at chapter 4—in it, I talk about some of my experiences with these treatments and I ask some of New York City's top dermatologists to weigh in with their thoughts. There's great info that will help you decide what to do. Just remember to stay true to yourself and what makes YOU special.

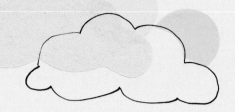

How do you personally deal with stress? Obviously you're doing something right because you look so good and have such a happy, healthy mental outlook.

Stress comes in many shapes and sizes and wears many hats. So you have to have a variety of ways to cope with it—no, not just cope, THRIVE!

Stress is a fact of life, so you have to be ready with a response. Stress wreaks havoc on your immune system; during stressful times, it's even more important to make sure you're getting your B vitamins, exercising to release serotonin (the feel-good hormone), and smiling as much as possible. Trust me, just putting your lips in a smiling position releases so many feel-good hormones that you will feel an immediate surge. Stress will knot you up, so release the stress with yoga and breathing exercises—exhale the stress, inhale peace. Being surrounded by people in a crowded yoga class is very calming to me. I feel like I am in the rainbow of their auras. I know that sounds esoteric, but you really can feel the good vibes and good intentions, and it's lovely! And whenever possible, I also try to get a massage to help me relax.

Meditation is great for centering yourself, but sometimes I'm too hyper to just stop like that. So I decompress with a camera in hand, and I take a walk to look for beauty. I love the beach and the woods and am lucky to live by both, but I can find beauty in any city too. I see beauty everywhere, and I am in awe and overwhelmed with gratitude that flowers exist, that leaves crunch, that birds sing, and that clouds grace the sky in an ever-changing art show of both sculptures and paintings! Looking for beauty fills up my heart and soul, makes me less stressed, and heals whatever is hurting. Being in nature is where I find my peace and feel so alive and thriving. I hope you're still smiling!

I do enjoy exercising, but I still have a hard time getting on that elliptical every day! Any advice?

I hear you! But I have to say that I don't think *anyone* would want to get on that elliptical EVERY day. The first thing I would suggest is adding variety. Can you get outside on some days, go for a walk or a jog? Or take a bike ride? If not, and the elliptical is your mainstay exercise, add music (always inspiring!) and mix up your routine. Maybe just do ten minutes on the elliptical, then jump off and do a plank. (Keep track of how long you can hold it and start a competition with yourself. I like to see improvement; it keeps me going.) Add some push-ups, then jump back on the elliptical for another ten, this time with weights in your hands, and see what you can do at a slower speed while working your arms. Even just two-pound weights in each hand—lifting your arms over your head, then out to the side—will increase your heart rate and work your upper body as you burn calories. Check out chapter 3 for more ideas to spice up your exercise menu!

And when I get lazy about exercising, I think about my goals—both short- and long-term. My short-term goals focus on the things I want to be able to do every day. I want to be in good enough shape that I can play with my kids—ski with them, jump on the paddleboard, just be able to have fun and do the things they want to do. And I also try to stay focused on my long-term goal of remaining strong so I can stay independent and healthy into my later years. Like all of us, when life gets hectic, the first thing that goes is my time to exercise. But without exercise, I'm done for. My weight creeps up and my body doesn't feel as good. So I've learned that making that time for me is so important. Invest in your health—it's your greatest wealth!

After fifty, are you supposed to give up the style you love and become conservative?

NOOOOOOOO! You are never supposed to give up your style. It's an expression of who you are. You make your own rules! You decide! If we were all the same, following all the same rules, what fun would that be? As Coco Chanel once said, "In order to be irreplaceable, one must always be different."

Of course the world is constantly judging, and "appropriate attire" can be important for certain occasions. But even that should not be determined purely by your age. If you are happy with a look, that should be all that matters. Some people are just meant to be eccentric and wonderfully original. And if that's you, then it's my pleasure to make your acquaintance!

As someone who is still fairly young, how can I prevent my skin from aging?

I have one word for you: SUNSCREEN! Wearing it every day is the single most important thing you can do to keep your skin looking young. And every dermatologist I've ever talked to agrees. You need to wear sunscreen every day, no matter what, even in winter, even on cloudy days. The ultraviolet rays from the sun (as well as the infrared radiation that comes from anything that emits heat—like stoves, computers, hair dryers) break down the collagen in your skin. And that's why skin gets saggy and wrinkled as you get older. Too much sun also causes skin to overproduce melanin, and that can lead to dark spots and uneven skin tone. You could save yourself a fortune on antiaging products and procedures down the road if you're really diligent with your sunscreen now!

Staying in shape and maintaining a healthy weight will help in the long run too. If your weight yo-yos up and down, that can stretch out your skin and lead to extra sagging. And don't forget to wear a supportive sports bra for all those high-impact activities!

No matter how much rest I get or what cover-up I use, I cannot get rid of my dark undereye circles! What can I do?

Dark circles can be really tricky to deal with, and as you've recognized, they don't necessarily have anything to do with whether or not you've gotten a good night's sleep. One thing I've noticed that does help is drinking LOTS of water. Some of that darkness is because you're seeing blood through the skin, and that's exacerbated by being dehydrated. Also, look for undereye creams that can help. Certain ingredients (like caffeine) can immediately firm the undereye skin and reduce bags, while optical diffusers can blur and blend away the look of darkness. My **REFOCUS Undereye Treatment** has rose extract, which helps eliminate the dark circles.

When it comes to covering them with concealer, sometimes it takes more than one color. I start with a light yellow tone applied with a brush on the area that has the most darkness. Then I use a more standard undereye concealer applied with my finger—the body heat will sort of melt them into each other. I add a sunnier color just at the edges where the concealer blends into my face and finish with a touch of powder just on the darkest area (NOT all over under the eye, because I don't want it to cake up). The **Alcone** concealer palettes are great for eliminating circles—find more details on page 130.

Do you know any products or treatments that tighten the skin on the neck?

Yes, the **UPLIFT Firming Neck & Décolleté Treatment** from my **Christie Brinkley Authentic Skincare** line can help! Honestly, I've seen really great results using it. The active ingredients work to increase collagen production to help firm skin. For more dramatic results, there are also some great treatments your dermatologist can do—such as **Thermage** and **Ultherapy**, devices that stimulate the production of new collagen over time. Check out chapter 4 for more details on these procedures.

What are your postmenopause beauty secrets? I am battling thinning hair, dark spots, dry skin, etc.

Eating right, avoiding stress (is that even possible?), and taking a supplement designed to help your hair retain its fullness and shine (such as **Bio-Sil**) are all important, but the fastest and easiest way to deal with thinning hair is to add extensions. They are so easy to use—just snap them on in three seconds for instant youthful fullness! (See chapter 6 for some step-by-step instructions on using hair extensions.) If you have spots where you can see through to the scalp that you are sensitive about, you can fill them in with a spray like **Rita Hazan Root Concealer** or **Giorgio Armani Eye & Brow Maestro** (men in show biz are familiar with this quick trick). Another way to add fullness is with a dry shampoo or thickening spray. My favorite is **Oribe Dry Texturizing Spray**—use before adding a clip-on extension for great grip. Some doctors may recommend a treatment like **Rogaine**, which works as long as you keep using it. Your doctor can also prescribe **Latisse**, which really works to thicken eyelashes that can also diminish after menopause. For more volumizing ideas (including how your diet can make your hair look fuller), go to chapter 6.

Dark spots aren't specifically related to menopausal changes, but often show up coincidentally around that time. That's because they are the result of all our years of sun exposure. You can still prevent new ones from developing (at any age) by using a good, broad-spectrum sunscreen every day. To fade ones you already have, you can try lotions and serums with ingredients such as vitamin C, soy, or peptides. (I like **Dr. Brandt Light Years Away Whitening Essence**.) Laser treatments from your dermatologist can also target dark spots, breaking up the pigment to make it disappear. But you must be diligent with sunscreen after the treatment or the spots will reappear.

And as for dry skin, it's not your imagination that your face and your body get dry and flaky faster than they used to. That's because as we get older, our sebaceous glands slow down their oil production. And less oil means skin that's easily dehydrated (which can make fine lines start to look like deep wrinkles). The key is to switch to more emollient products for your skin. The stuff you used in your thirties (or even your forties) might not work for you in your fifties and sixties. A moisturizer that contains hyaluronic acid or glycerin can help. Those ingredients are humectants, which means they help draw moisture into the skin and trap it there.

Do you take hormone replacement therapy, and what do you think about that subject?

I have not done any hormone replacement therapy, or even really researched much about it, because I honestly had zero menopause symptoms. Well, apart from my hair being less full, and what was that other thing? Oh yeah, forgetfulness! But I do consider myself very lucky. (Don't hate me! I'm sure the rest of the symptoms are around the corner.) I know that many women suffer from a lot of really unpleasant symptoms during this transition. All I can say is that you should talk to your doctor and do your own research on what you think might be best. Everyone is different, so I don't think there is one simple answer to this question. If there is one, please let me know—as you know, you can always reach me on Instagram!

Can you address sagging, aging skin on upper arms, thighs, and knees?

I could write a whole chapter about this problem on the saggy part under my upper arm...plenty of room there!

Joking aside, it is, unfortunately, a somewhat inevitable effect of getting older that skin will lose some of its elasticity. If you've been really, really diligent with sun protection all your life, your skin will be in better shape. But if you've spent your life playing in the sun (as I did and still do!), you'll probably notice that your skin's not quite as smooth and taut as it used to be. Staying at a healthy weight and keeping your muscles firm and fit are your best bets for beating sagging. (Try adding some heavier weights to your arm workout to build muscle and reduce sagging.) But what to do if the sagging is a fait accompli? Well, I am happy to report that there are some treatments your dermatologist can provide that will help to stimulate your own collagen and tighten skin (like the TriPollar Apollo and Ultherapy). Maybe not back to its former, firmer glory, but enough so you will see some improvement. Read more about this topic in chapter 4. And if all else fails, be on the lookout for cute shrugs and long-sleeved sweaters you can toss on!

What are some tips for working out when you're completely out of shape and over-whelmed by the idea of trying to exercise?

I know it can be hard—especially if you are out of shape and you feel weak, or have pain. Your goals and your reality may seem miles apart. But if you really want to change something, something has to change. You are not going to get any stronger or fitter if you don't start somewhere.

I think a good strategy for you might be to start with several mini sessions throughout the day, right in your own home. For example: Can you do a push-up on your knees? How many? If the answer is two at eight o'clock in the morning, see if you can do three at noon and three again before dinner. Keep tabs on your progress and set small goals. You will marvel at how quickly your body will respond. Push-ups, planks, squats, light hand weights, and stretch bands are all options to try at home. And check out chapter 3 for some of my favorite "multi-taskercises" that you can do during the course of your daily routine. Look for opportunities throughout the day when you can walk more—even a few ten-minute walks daily can help build your endurance and keep your heart healthy.

I also find it really helpful to surround myself with healthy, positive, inspiring people and images. I might stick a photo of someone I think looks particularly great on my fridge to remind me not to nibble mindlessly. And put a lot of healthy people on your Facebook and Instagram feeds. Seeing their posts and photos of fresh, healthy food and fun workouts will help keep you inspired and motivated.

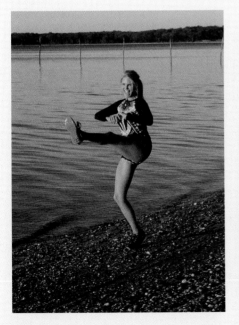 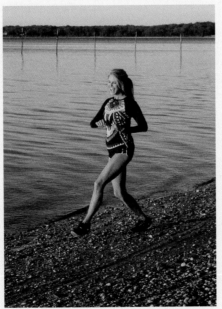 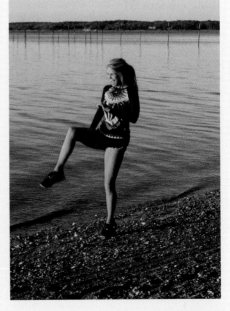

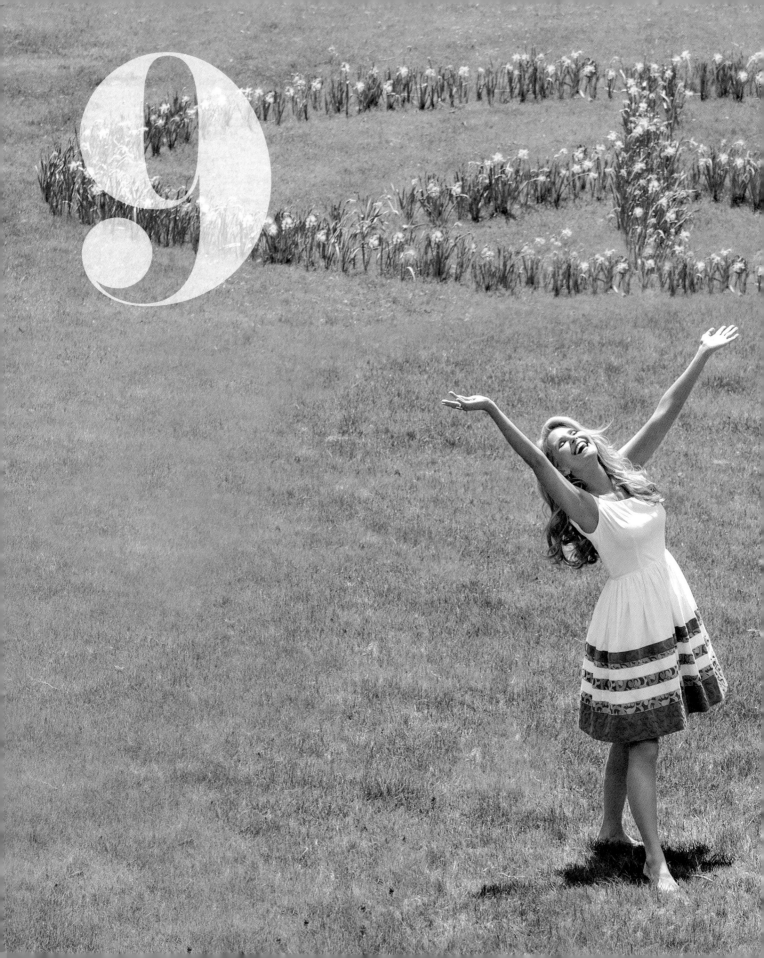

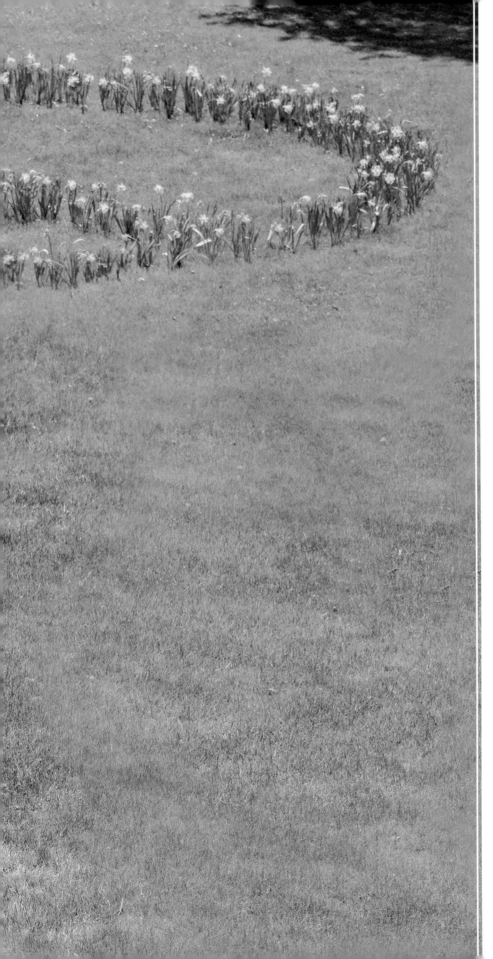

THE BEAUTY OF GIVING BACK

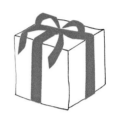

Each time you reach out to help, you are exercising your heart muscles in the most beautiful way.

One of the practices that I believe helps me to maintain my positive outlook is reaching out to help the causes I believe in. And there are so MANY worthy and important causes out there! Taking care of our earth, supporting organic and local farmers, empowering our children, and protecting animals—these are just a few of the things I'm passionate about. When I became a mom, that's when I really became an activist. I started seeing the world not just how it is now, but how it will be for my kids. So I want to feel like I've done everything in my power to leave them a world that's a better place. In this chapter you'll find a guide to all of my favorite causes and organizations. But I would also encourage you to seek out ones that really speak to you and represent the things that are important in your life.

Giving back and making a difference are the quickest ways to buff up your inner beauty. And as you've heard me say numerous times throughout this book, that is such a key component of true beauty. If you've read this far, you've already learned all the tricks you need to enhance your physical beauty (great skin, flawless makeup, amazing hair)—but all that will be empty without spending equal effort to enhance your inner beauty.

The other reason I believe that giving back is a beautiful thing to do is that it always fills me with gratitude—for what I have, how I'm able to help, and for all the other beautiful people out there in the world striving to make a difference. And gratitude is another one of those positive emotions that will be reflected back on you to make you more beautiful. Don't you just love how that works?!

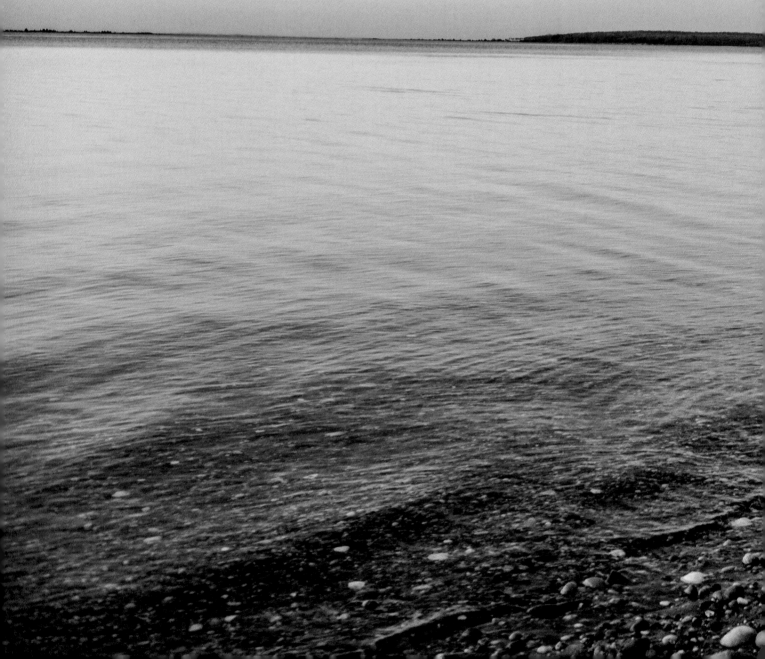

"*Just remember you're blessed beyond measure. Every day is a day you should treasure.*"

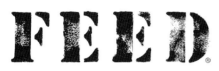

feedprojects.com

Founded by Lauren Bush Lauren in 2007, the organization sells products (like its original FEED bag) that literally help feed the world. Each product is stamped with a number that relates to a measurable donation—for example, the original burlap FEED bag is stamped with a "1" because the proceeds from it will feed one child for one school year.

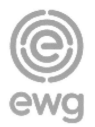

ewg.org

The EWG (Environmental Working Group) provides consumers with research on toxins and environmental health, food and agriculture, and water and energy. Each year they put out a list of the "Dirty Dozen," the most pesticide-laden produce, and their Skin Deep database helps sort through which beauty products are safest to use.

glwd.org

God's Love We Deliver was founded in 1985 when one woman began delivering food on her bicycle to a man dying from AIDS. The organization now cooks 4,600 meals each weekday, delivering them, free of charge, to clients who are too ill to shop and cook for themselves in all five boroughs of New York City, Newark, and Hudson County, New Jersey.

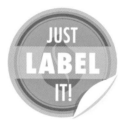

justlabelit.org

As this book went to press, there was still no Federal law mandating manufacturers to label foods that contain GMOs. That means that there's no way of knowing what you're buying, eating, and feeding your family. Hopefully, JLI—and all of the organizations that are already on board with its mission—will succeed in changing that soon.

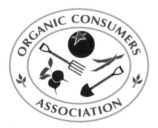

organicconsumers.org

If you're interested in issues regarding organic food, GMOs, and other food safety topics, check out the OCA. It's a great place to find up-to-date information on these issues as well as ways you can get involved.

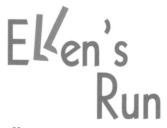

ellensrun.org

This is an annual event where I live on Long Island, and the race helps support the Ellen Hermanson Breast Center at Southampton Hospital and raise money for the Ellen Hermanson Foundation, which educates and supports women in the community who are facing breast cancer.

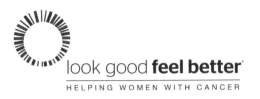

lookgoodfeelbetter.org

This wonderful organization brings together beauty professionals to help women who are going through cancer treatment. They provide group programs that teach women tricks for coping with appearance-related side effects of cancer treatments, plus the support to help them maintain their self-confidence.

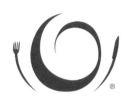

sustainabletable.org

This is another great resource for staying informed about food issues and ways you can work to make a difference in how our food system operates.

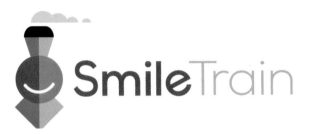

smiletrain.org

Every year, over 170,000 children around the world are born with a cleft lip and/or palate—many of them to families who are unable to afford surgery to correct it. Smile Train provides free cleft repair surgeries to those in need while helping to train local doctors. This makes it possible for a child born with a cleft to eat, breathe, speak properly, and smile.

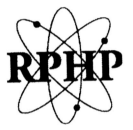

radiation.org

I turn to this organization for up-to-date information and the latest scientific research on the effects of low-level radiation on our health—especially its link to cancer and childhood diseases.

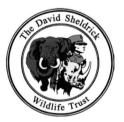

sheldrickwildlifetrust.org

The plight of African elephants is a cause close to my heart. This organization runs programs to rescue orphan elephants and also antipoaching projects to help save these amazing animals and their natural habitats.

GLOBAL
SECURITY
INSTITUTE

gsinstitute.org

This group works toward a goal of international security by promoting nuclear arms control, nonproliferation, and disarmament.

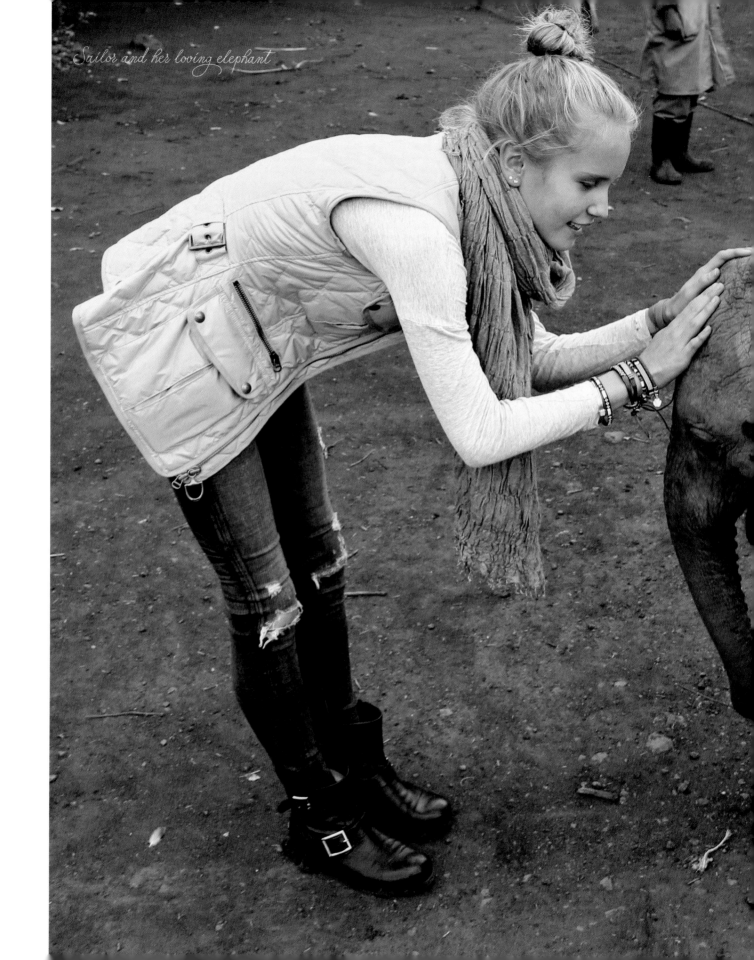

Sailor and her loving elephant

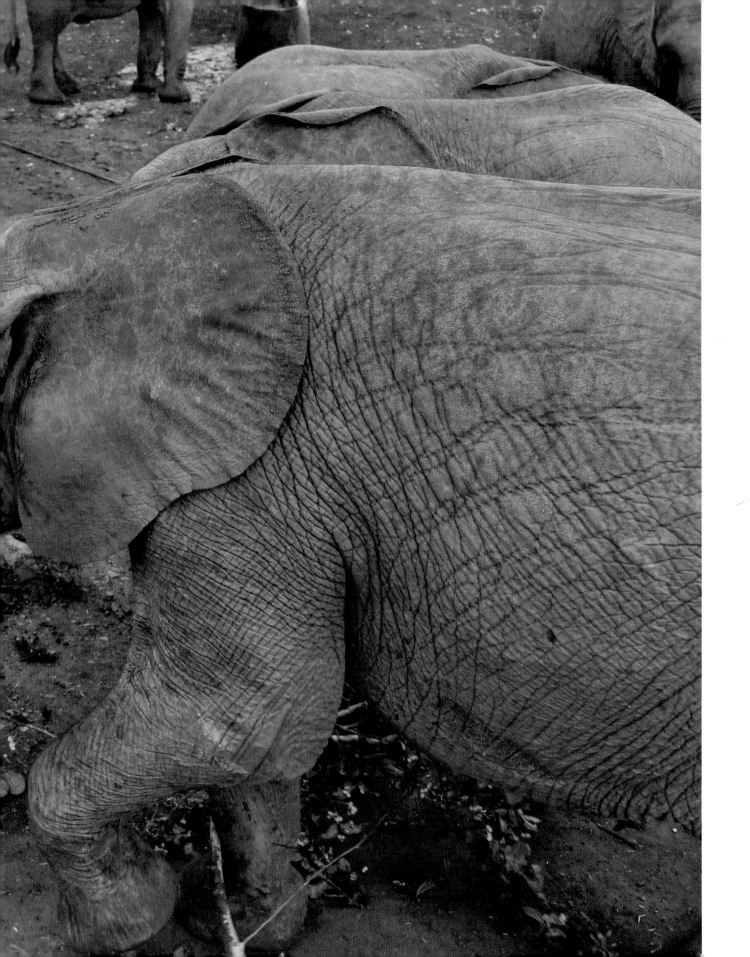

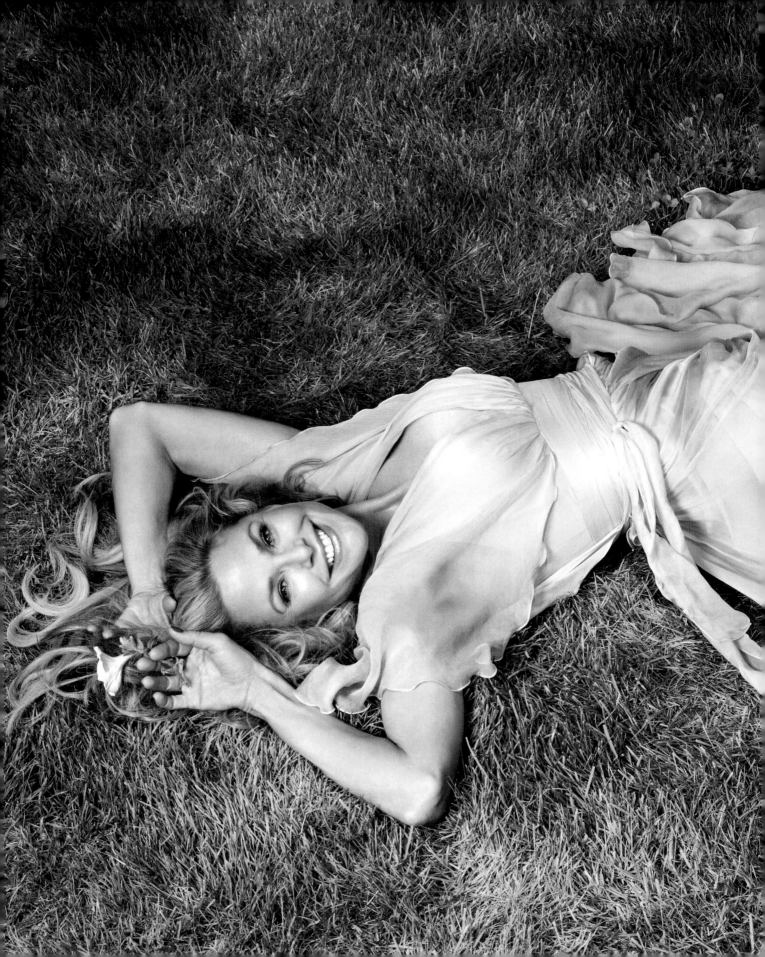

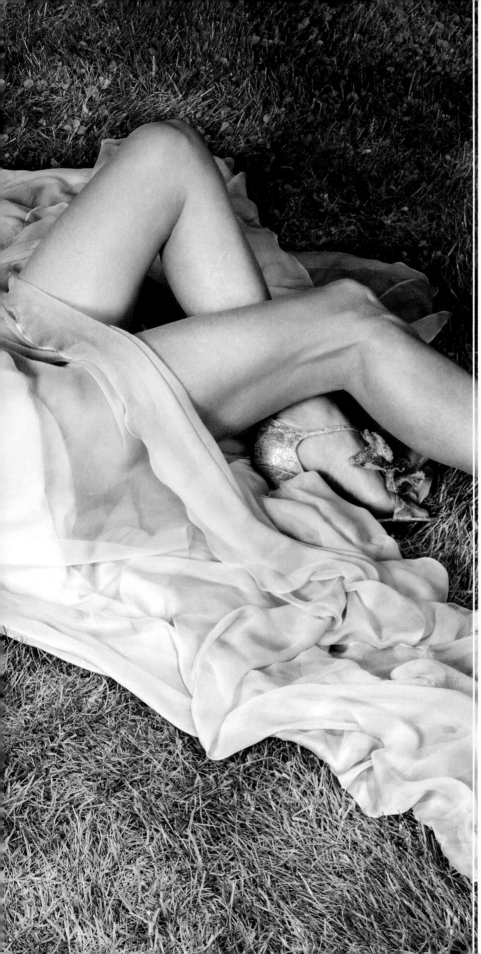

RESOURCE GUIDE

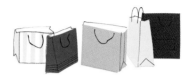

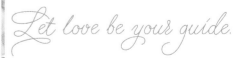

Let love be your guide.

1

Pepsodent toothpaste
www.pepsodent.in

Crest Pro-Health Whitening
toothpaste
www.crest.com

Oral-B toothbrushes
www.oralb.com

2

Maine Coast Sea Vegetables
www.seaveg.com

Ancient Harvest Gluten-Free Quinoa
Ancient Harvest Quinoa Hot Flakes
Cereal
Supergrain Pasta
www.ancientharvest.com

truRoots Ancient Grain Pastas
www.truroots.com

Bio-K probiotics
www.biokplus.com

Living Intentions
Salad Booster
www.livingintentions.com

3

Ari Weller, physical therapist
www.philosofit.com
15 Lumber Lane
East Hampton, NY 11937
631-527-5070

Sinead Fitzgibbon, physical therapist
www.muvPT.com/about

MobilityWOD Supernova
massage ball
www.roguefitness.com

Total Gym
www.totalgym.com

4

BioSil advanced collagen
generators
www.biosilusa.com

Activz
www.activz.com

Proactiv
www.proactiv.com

Elizabeth Arden Eight Hour
Cream Skin Protectant
www.elizabetharden.com

Neutrogena Wet Skin Sunscreen Spray,
Broad Spectrum SPF 85+
www.neutrogena.com

Christie Brinkley Authentic Skincare
www.christiebrinkleyauthenticskin
care.com

Jergens BB Body Perfecting
Skin Cream
www.jergens.com

NARS Pure Radiant Tinted Moisturizer,
Broad Spectrum SPF 30
www.narscosmetics.com

Laura Mercier Tinted Moisturizer,
Broad Spectrum SPF 20 for face
www.lauramercier.com

Clarins Extra-Firming Body Cream
www.clarinsusa.com

Evian Mineral Water Spray
www.evianspray.com

Laura Mercier Almond
Coconut Milk
Soufflé Body Crème
www.lauramercier.com

Robert Anolik, MD
www.laserskinsurgery.com
317 East 34th Street
New York, NY 10016
212-686-7306

Doris Day, MD
www.myclearskin.com
10 East 70th Street
New York, NY 10021
212-772-0740

Ellen Gendler, MD
www.ellengendler.com
1035 Fifth Avenue
New York, NY 10028
212-288-8222

5

Christie Brinkley Authentic
Skincare Close Up Instant Wrinkle
Reducer & Treatment
www.christiebrinkleyauthenticskin
care.com

Chanel Le Blanc de Chanel
Multi-Use Illuminating Base
www.chanel.com

Christie Brinkley Authentic
Skincare Refocus Eye + IR Defense
www.christiebrinkleyauthenticskin
care.com

Christie Brinkley Authentic
Skincare Recapture 360 + IR Defense
Anti-Aging Day Cream
www.christiebrinkleyauthenticskin
care.com

Kevyn Aucoin The Sensual
Skin Enhancer
www.kevynaucoin.com

3LAB Perfect BB Cream SPF 40
www.3lab.com

Giorgio Armani Maestro
Octinoxate Sunscreen Fusion Makeup,
Broad Spectrum SPF 15
www.giorgioarmanibeauty-usa.com

Kevyn Aucoin Foundation Brush
www.kevynaucoin.com

Make Up For Ever
Aqua Brow
www.makeupforever.com

Make Up For Ever
Angled Eyebrow Brush
www.makeupforever.com

Laura Mercier
Illuminating Powder
www.lauramercier.com

Kevyn Aucoin Super Soft
Buff Powder Brush
www.kevynaucoin.com

By Terry Hyaluronic Blush
www.byterry.com

Clarins Moisture
Replenishing Lip Balm
www.clarinsusa.com

Kevyn Aucoin Eyelash Curler
www.kevynaucoin.com

Make Up For Ever Aqua
Matic Waterproof
Glide-On Eye Shadow
www.makeupforever.com

Lancôme Le Crayon Khôl
www.lancome-usa.com

Make Up For Ever Smoky
Extravagant Mascara
www.makeupforever.com

Freedom System
Eye Shadow
www.inglotusa.com

NARS Sheer Matte Foundation
www.narscosmetics.com

Bobbi Brown Long-Wear
Even Finish Foundation
www.bobbibrowncosmetics.com

Urban Decay Naked
Basics Palette
www.urbandecay.com

Sonia Kashuk for Target
eye shadow brush
www.target.com

Bobbi Brown lip pencil
www.bobbibrowncosmetics.com

Make Up For Ever
Aqua Eyes eyeliner
www.makeupforever.com

Kiss i-Envy Short
Black Individual Lashes
and Strip Lash Adhesive
www.ienvybykiss.com

Lancôme Lip Lover
www.lancome-usa.com

NARS Lip Gloss
www.narscosmetics.com

Christie Brinkley Authentic
Skincare creamy scrub
www.christiebrinkleyauthenticskin
care.com

St. Ives Fresh Skin
Apricot Scrub
www.stives.com

Olay Regenerist
Regenerating Lotion
with Sunscreen
Broad Spectrum SPF 50
www.olay.com

Laura Mercier
Brow Powder
Laura Mercier Brow Pencil
www.lauramercier.com

Chanel Le Sourcil de
Chanel Perfect Brows
www.chanel.com

Lancôme Le Crayon Poudre
brow pencils
www.lancome-usa.com

Giorgio Armani Eye
& Brow Maestro
www.giorgioarmanibeauty-usa.com

NARS Lip Gloss
www.narscosmetics.com

MAC Lip Pencil
www.maccosmetics.com

Alcone makeup sponges
www.alconeco.com

Bobbi Brown's customizable palettes
www.bobbibrowncosmetics.com

Inglot Cosmetics Freedom
System palettes
www.inglotusa.com

Viseart palettes
www.viseart.com

YSL Touche Éclat
www.yslbeautyus.com

Sandy Linter, makeup artist
www.sandylinter.com
Follow her on Instagram
@sandylinter

Lancôme Le Corrector Pro Concealer Kit
www.lancome-usa.com

Vicks VapoRub
www.vicks.com

Dr. Gendler's Foot
Recovery Cream
www.ellengendler.com

Dermasil Labs Pharmaceutical
Research Dry Skin
Treatment Original Lotion
www.dermasillabs.com

Denise Markey, makeup artist
www.abtp.com
Follow her on Instagram
@denisemarkey

Kryolan Dermacolor
Mini Concealer
Palette from Alcone
www.us.kryolan.com

Three Custom Color Specialists
Clarifier eye pencil
www.threecustom.com

Moyra Mulholland, makeup artist
www.bryanbantry.com

Physicians Formula Eye Booster 2-in-1
Lash Boosting Eyeliner + Serum
www.physiciansformula.com

DuWop Lip Venom
www.shop.duwop.com

Rogaine
www.rogaine.com

Hair2wear extensions
www.hair2wear.com

Jen Atkin, hairstylist
www.jenatkin.com
Follow her on Instagram
@jenatkinhair

Aquis Essentials Hair Towel
www.aquis.com

Oribe Dry Texturizing Spray
www.oribe.com

Philip B Russian
Amber Imperial Insta-Thick
Hair Thickening & Finishing Spray
www.philipb.com

Maury Hopson, hairstylist
mhopson1@nyc.rr.com

Ceramicare Thermal
Vented brushes
www.amazon.com

Mitch Barry, hairstylist
www.bryanbantry.com

Sally Hershberger
Plump Up Collagen
Thickening Mist
www.sallyhershberger.com

Sharon Dorram,
hair colorist
www.sharondorram.com

Sally Hershberger Supreme
Lift Root Spray
www.sallyhershberger.com

Solano Supersolano
3300 xtralite hair dryer
www.solanopower.com

Oribe Grandiose Hair Plumping Mousse
Oribe Maximista Thickening Spray
www.oribe.com

Sun-In spray-in hair lightener
www.sun-in.com

Terax Life Drops
www.teraxhaircare.com

Prell shampoo
www.prell.com

L'Oréal Paris Elnett Satin Hairspray
Extra Strong Hold (Unscented)
www.lorealparisusa.com

Rita Hazan Root Concealer
www.ritahazan.com

Mason Pearson hairbrush
www.masonpearson.co.uk

Denman hairbrush
www.denmanbrushus.com

Kevin Mancuso, hairstylist
www.kevinmancuso.com
Follow him on Instagram
@kevinmancusonyc

Super Million Hair
Enhancement Fibers
www.smhair.com

Nexxus Emergencée
Reconstructing Treatment
www.nexxus.com

Wayne Scot Lukas, stylist
Follow him on Instagram
@wslukastyle

Commando Classic Thong
www.wearcommando.com

Trust Your Thinstincts by Spanx
www.spanx.com

OnGossamer Sheer Bliss T-Shirt Bra
www.ongossamer.com

Gossard Superboost Plunge Bra
www.gossardusa.com

Wacoal Red Carpet Strapless Bra
www.wacoal-america.com

Le Mystère Sculptural Strapless Bra
www.lemystere.com

OnGossamer mesh bikini and brief
www.ongossamer.com

Hanky Panky thongs
www.hankypanky.com

Fogal stockings
www.fogal.com

Wolford stockings
www.wolfordshop.com

Phillip Bloch, stylist
www.phillipbloch.com

MAC Studio Face and
Body Foundation
www.maccosmetics.com

Kérastase Resistance
Ciment Thermique
www.kerastase-usa.com

Oribe Gel Sérum Radiance,
Magic and Hold
www.oribe.com

KeVita Sparkling Probiotic Drink
www.kevita.com

Christie Brinkley Authentic
Skincare Uplift Firming
Neck & Décolleté Treatment
www.christiebrinkleyauthenticskin
care.com

Latisse
www.latisse.com

Dr. Brandt Light Years
Away Whitening Essence
www.drbrandtskincare.com

Photo Credits

trip, (3) Uli Rose, (4) Copyright Timothy White 2015, (5) Christie Brinkley archive—at work in Dermachelier's studio, (6) Christie Brinkley archive—Mexico, (7) Christie Brinkley archive—Turks and Caicos Islands; **pages 12–13:** Anna Gunselman; **page 14:** Anna Gunselman; **page 15:** Paul Mesher; **page 16,** *left:* Christie Brinkley archive—with Alexa and my mom, *right:* Anna Gunselman; **page 17,** *clockwise from top left:* (1) Christie Brinkley archive—with my mom, (2) Christie Brinkley archive—with my sonshine, Jack, (3) Christie Brinkley archive—Africa, (4) Christie

Page 3: Andrew Macpherson/CPi Syndication; **page 5:** Christie Brinkley archive; **page 8,** *clockwise from top center:* (1) Courtesy *People* magazine, (2) Motion Picture Artwork © 2015 Courtesy of Warner Bros. Ent., Inc. All rights reserved. (3) Joseph Marzullo/Wenn.com, (4) ©1991 Todd Kaplan, (5) Christie Brinkley archive—Paris; **page 9,** *clockwise from top left:* (1) photo by Andrew Eccles/PLAYBILL cover courtesy of Playbill, Inc., Use of "Chicago The Musical" courtesy of The Chicago Limited Partnership. All rights reserved, (2) Alex Chatelain, (3) John G. Zimmerman/ *Sports Illustrated*, (4) John G. Zimmerman/ *Sports Illustrated*, (5) Walter Iooss, Jr./*Sports Illustrated*, (6) Reprinted with permission of Simon & Schuster, Inc. from *Christie Brinkley's Outdoor Beauty and Fitness Book*, by Christie Brinkley. All rights reserved; **Page 10,** *top left:* Walter Iooss, Jr./*Sports Illustrated*, *bottom left:* Courtesy of *Harper's Bazaar*, Hearst Communications, Inc., *center:* Courtesy of *Harper's Bazaar*, Hearst Communications, Inc., *top right:* Christie Brinkley archive—billboard Times Square, Use of "Chicago The Muscial" courtesy of The Chicago Limited Partnership. All rights reserved. *bottom right:* Christie Brinkley archive—Morocco; **Page 11,** *clockwise from top left:* (1) Courtesy of *Harper's Bazaar*, Hearst Communications, Inc., (2) Christie Brinkley archive—*Sports Illustrated*

Brinkley archive—with my "two little ones," Sailor and Jack; **page 18,** *both images,* Anna Gunselman; **page 19:** Christie Brinkley archive—Lucky House, Parrot Cay, Turks and Caicos Islands; **pages 20–21:** Anna Gunselman; **pages 22–23:** Anna Gunselman; **page 24:** Anna Gunselman; **page 25,** *from top left:* (1) Christie Brinkley archive, (2) Christie Brinkley archive, (3) Anna Gunselman; **page 27:** Anna Gunselman; **page 28:** Paul Mesher, **page 29:** Anna Gunselman; **page 32:** Anna Gunselman; **pages 34–35,** *both photos,* Anna Gunselman; **page 36,** *both photos:* Anna Gunselman; **pages 37–53:** Marcus Donates/ Beast Media; **pages 54–57:** Christie Brinkley archive; **page 58:** Anna Gunselman; **page 60:** Anna Gunselman; **pages 62–63:** Anna Gunselman; **page 65:** Anna Gunselman; **pages 66–67,** *left:* Photo by Andrew Eccles, Use of "Chicago The Musical" courtesy of The Chicago Limited Partnership. All rights reserved, *far right:* Jeremy Daniel, Use of "Chicago The Musical" courtesy of The Chicago Limited Partnership. All rights reserved; **pages 68–79:** Anna Gunselman; **pages 80–81:** Anna Gunselman; **page 82:** Mindy Moak; **page 87:** Anna Gunselman; **pages 88–92** *(photos of Christie Brinkley):* Anna Gunselman; **pages 94–95,** *left, top to bottom:* (1) Michael Benabib, (2) Stephen Scott Gross Photography, (3) Courtesy of Ellen Gendler, MD, *right:* Anna Gunselman; **page 98:** Christie Brinkley archive; **pages 100–101:** Anna Gunselman; **pages 102–103:** Anna Gunselman: **page 104:** Paul Mesher; **pages 106–107,** *all covers:* courtesy of the Francesco Scavullo Foundation, the estate of Francesca Scavullo & courtesy of *Harper's Bazaar*, Hearst Communications, Inc.;

pages 108–114: Anna Gunselman; page 116, *top:* Christie Brinkley archive, *bottom:* Anna Gunselman; page 117, *both images:* Anna Gunselman; pages 118–119: Anna Gunselman; page 122: Anna Gunselman; page 124: Christie Brinkley archive; page 125: Photo by Michael Thompson; page 126, *clockwise from top:* (1) Courtesy *People* magazine, (2) Paul Mesher, (3) Paul Mesher; page 127, *all three covers:* Courtesy of Francesco Scavullo Foundation, the estate of Francesca Scavullo & courtesy of *Harper's Bazaar*, Hearst Communications, Inc.; page 128: Paul Mesher, page 129, *all images:* Christie Brinkley archive; page 130: Photo by Andrew Eccles; Use of "Chicago The Muscial" courtesy of The Chicago Limited Partnership. All rights reserved. page 131: Christie Brinkley archive; pages 132-133, *center:* Anna Gunselman; page 132, *bottom right:* Rico Puhlmann—Rico Puhlmann Archives; page 133, *top right:* Anna Gunselman, *bottom left:* Photo by Kate Orne/Cover courtesy of *Hamptons* magazine; pages 134–135: Ruven Afanador; page 136, *left:* Ron Galella/Getty Images, *right:* Patrick Demarchelier; page 137, *clockwise from top left:* (1) Christie Brinkley archive, (2) Courtesy of the Francesco Scavullo Foundation, the estate of Francesca Scavullo, (3) Patrick Demarchelier, (4) Anna Gunselman, (5) © John G. Zimmerman, *center:* Images Press/Getty Images; pages 138–139, *center:* Anna Gunselman;

page 141, *all three images:* Anna Gunselman; pages 142–143: Copyright Timothy White 2015; pages 144–145, *center:* Christie Brinkley archive; page 145: Jon Kopaloff/Getty Images; page 146, *left:* Christie Brinkley archive—Ali/Holmes fight, Las Vegas; *right:* Christie Brinkley archive—St. Barts; page 147, *top:* Christie Brinkley archive, *bottom:* Christie Brinkley archive; page 148: Erin Baiano/photographer; page 150: Courtesy of the Francesco Scavullo Foundation, the estate of Francesca Scavullo; page 151: Anna Gunselman;

pages 152–153: Photograph by Bruce Weber for Barneys NY. Copyright Bruce Weber; page 154, *clockwise from top left:* (1) Christie Brinkley archive—Morocco, (2) Christie Brinkley archive—Morocco, (3) Christie Brinkley archive, South Africa, (4) Christie Brinkley archive—Japan, (5) Christie Brinkley archive—Morocco, (6) Christie Brinkley archive—Morocco, *center:* Christie Brinkley archive—France; page 155: Christie Brinkley archive; page 156, *clockwise from top left:* (1) Christie Brinkley archive—Texas, (2) Christie Brinkley archive—Marrakech, (3) Christie Brinkley archive—Texas, (4) Christie Brinkley archive—Marrakech, (5) Don Shugart photography, (6) Christie Brinkley archive—Martha's Vineyard; page 157, *clockwise from top left:* (1) Christie Brinkley archive—trophy belt, (2) Paul Mesher, (3) Anna Gunselman, (4) Christie Brinkley archive—Marrakech, (5) Courtesy

of *Harper's Bazaar*, Hearst Communications, Inc., (6) Christie Brinkley archive, *center:* Christie Brinkley archive—Texas; page 158: Felipe Ramales; page 160: Sailor Brinkley-Cook; page 161: Anna Gunselman; page 162: Christie Brinkley archive; page 163: Christie Brinkley archive; page 164, *left:* Cindy Ord/Getty Images, *right:* Axelle/Bauer-Griffin/Getty Images; page 165, *left:* Stephen Lovekin/Getty Images, *center:* Simon James/Getty Images, *right:* Gregory Allen; page 167, *left:* Ash Gupta, *right:* *New York Daily News* archive/Getty Images; pages 168–169: Anna Gunselman; pages 170–171: Anna Gunselman; page 172: Ash Gupta; page 183, *all images:* Anna Gunselman; pages 184–185: Anna Gunselman; pages 186–187: Anna Gunselman; pages 190–191: Christie Brinkley archive; pages 192–193: Photo by Kate Orne; page 200: Anna Gunselman, pages 206–207: Anna Gunselman; page 208: Christie Brinkley archive.

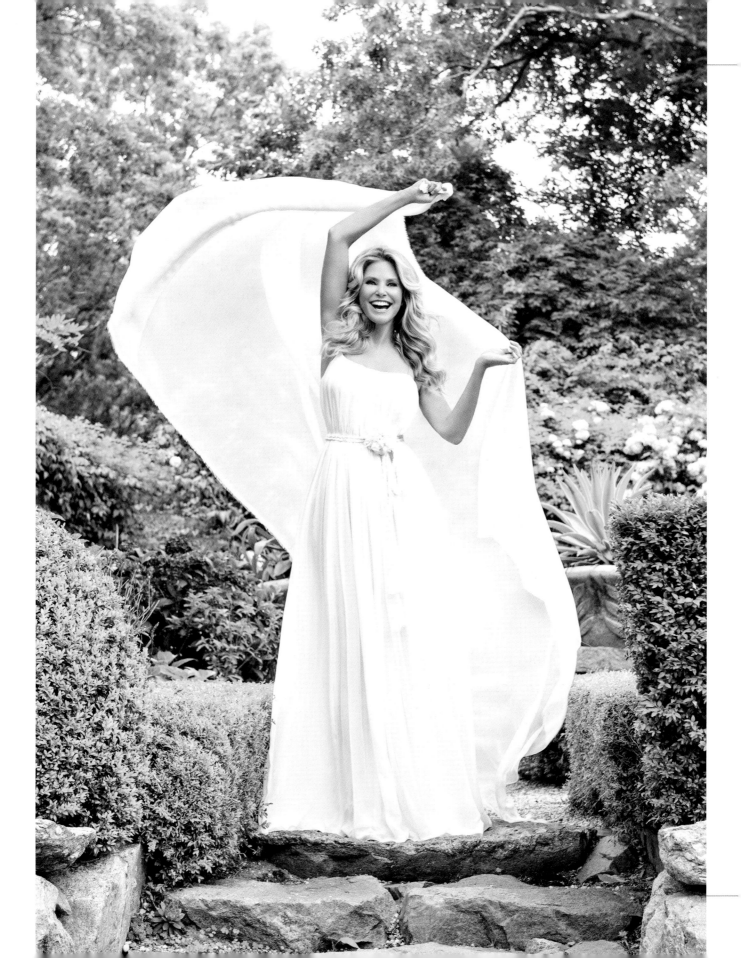

Acknowledgments

I want to thank my wonderful team. I am so lucky to have you all, because having a team means we get to share the blame...LOL! The first ones I'm going to blame are my book agents Brian Dubin and **Dan Strone;** and my editor, **Karen Murgolo** from Grand Central, who, despite never having met me, trusted me with this opportunity! I also want to acknowledge and thank every hair and makeup artist I've ever worked with. Your beautiful artistry helped me continue to work all these years, and for that I am so grateful. To all the photographers I've worked with—thank you for your talent and for always showing me in the best light. To the late and great **Eileen and Jerry Ford,** for introducing me to all the special people in our industry. Special mention to **Chef Gabi,** for creating the recipes in this book that taste so good, and to **Sally Wadyka** and **Bonnie Siegler,** for their good taste! Without your special guidance, expertise, and talent, this book wouldn't be as stylish, informative, or fun to look at. To **Paul Mesher,** for contributing his many skills throughout this process, and for his English accent that always adds some flair and elegance! To **Mindy Moak,** for her honest feedback on every chapter and for contributing photos of me with my kids that I cherish almost as much as our friendship. And, of course, to my kids, **Sailor, Alexa Ray, and Jack,** who keep me young by constantly filling my heart up with endless joy—as well as all the latest music!

Index

Activz, 85, 194
aerobic exercise, 61, 64, 72–73
alcohol, 83
almonds/almond milk, 30, 43, 49, 59
amaranth, 55
amino acids, 138
Anolik, Robert, 94, 96–97, 194
antiaging ingredients, for skin care, 87, 89
antiaging secrets, 124–25
antioxidants, 30–31, 32
apple cider vinegar, for sunburns, 91
apples, 30, 44, 61
applesauce, 59
arginine, 138, 175
arnica gel, 91
artichokes, 33, 56
Atkins, Jen, 144, 196
Aucoin, Kevyn, 106–7
avocados, 30, 37, 38, 40, 47, 50, 54, 174

bananas, 33, 37
Band Pulls, 71
Bandy, Way, 106
Barry, Mitch, 147, 196
bathing suits, 169
beans, 31, 42
bell peppers, 39, 41, 43, 52, 84
berries, 37, 84. *See also specific berries*
Bio-K probiotics, 29, 194
BioSil supplements, 85, 129, 181, 194
black tea bags, for eye puffiness, 91
Bloch, Phillip, 167, 197
blueberries, 30, 33, 84
blush, 112, 120, 124, 133
Bobbi Brown products, 117, 125, 195, 196
Botox, 17, 93, 95, 96, 98, 101, 176

Brandt, Frederic, 95, 181, 197
bras, 166, 197
Brazil nuts, 30, 85
broccoli, 30
butter, substitutes, 59
B vitamins, 138, 177

cabbage, 31, 44, 47
cacao powder, 59
calf raises, 128
calorie counting, 173
cardigans, 161
carnitine, 78
carrots, 40, 46, 48, 50, 84
Ceramicare Thermal Vented brushes, 146, 196
Chair Sit, 77
Chanel Le Sourcil de Chanel Perfect Brows, 123, 196
charitable giving, 186–89
cheekbones, 111, 112
cherries, dried tart, 31
chia seeds, 30
Chicago the Musical, 67, 72, 130, 147
chocolate substitutes, 59
Christie Brinkley Authentic Skincare products, 89, 108–9, 115, 180, 194, 195, 197
Clarins Moisture Replenishing Lip Balm, 112, 115, 195
Clear + Brilliant laser treatment, 93, 99
clothing. *See* fashion
coconut cream, 59
coconut oil, 59, 174
coconut sugar, 59
combs, 146
Commando Classic Thong, 166, 197

concealers, 109, 116, 121, 124, 127, 130
conditioners, 144, 149
cortisol, 78
cosmetic treatments, 92–101, 176
cranberries, dried, 33, 40, 42, 48
crunches, 68
curling irons, 141, 149

dairy substitutes, 59
dark chocolate, 31, 33
dark spots, 181
dates, 59
Day, Doris, 89, 94, 96–97, 194
"deny-iting" (deny dieting), 28, 60, 173
dermal fillers, 93, 96, 99, 176
dermatologists, finding, 100–101
desserts, 49, 53, 61
diet. *See* enlightened eating
dietary fiber, 31, 61
Dorram, Sharon, 148, 196
drinking water, 57, 61, 91
DuWop Lip Venom, 133, 196
Dynamic Plank, 70

eating plan, 60–61
"eating the rainbow," 32
eccentric exercises, 64, 70–71
edamame, 85
eggs, substitutes, 59
Elizabeth Arden Eight Hour Cream, 88, 194
Ellen's Run, 188
enlightened eating, 25–61. *See also* recipes
for beautiful hair, 138, 151, 174
for beautiful skin, 83–85

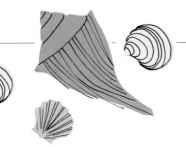

food sources, 26, 29
stocking your kitchen, 30–31
Environmental Working Group (EWG),
26, 88, 188
evening fashion look, 161
evening makeup look, 118
Evian Mineral Water Spray, 91, 121, 132,
194
exercise, 64–77. *See also* multi-taskercise
brain and benefits of, 78
daily habit of, 178
goals for, 73, 178, 183
injuries, 66–67
quick tips, 73
swim the sand, 72–73
top five at-home moves, 70–71
exfoliants (exfoliation), 87, 90, 96, 120
eyebrows, 123
cosmetic procedures, 98
everyday look, 111
overplucking, 120
thinning, 123, 175
eyelash curlers, 104, 113, 127
eyelashes, 113, 114, 116, 118, 124–25, 174
eye makeup, 127, 130, 132–33
evening look, 118
everyday look, 109, 111, 113, 114, 115
eyes look bigger, 174
office look, 116
eye puffiness, 91
eye shadow, 113, 115, 116, 123, 148

face lifts, 176
fashion, 155–69
the classics, 158–59
dressing your age, 168–69, 179
rules for dressing slimmer, 164–65

sources of inspiration for, 155–56
tricks for a night out, 161
fashion trends, 158, 162, 169
fat-reduction techniques, 99
Feed Projects, 188
fennel, 31, 33, 38
fermented foods, 31
fiber, 31, 61
fingernails, 129
fish and seafood, 26
Fitzgibbon, Sinead, 68, 73, 194
flax seeds, 30
food. *See* enlightened eating
food labeling, 29, 188
food substitutes, 58–59
foundation, 110, 116, 120, 130, 132, 133, 195
Freedom System Eye Shadow, 114, 115, 195
frowns (frowning), 17

garlic, 31
Gendler, Ellen, 94, 96–97, 194, 196
genetically modified organisms (GMOs),
26, 29, 188
Giorgio Armani products, 110, 115, 123,
175, 181, 195, 196
giving back, 186–89
Global Security Institute, 189
Glute Hinge, 71
goals, for exercise, 73, 178, 183
God's Love We Deliver, 188
grapes, 31, 33
gray hair, 148, 149
green tea, 84, 88

hair, 136–51
adding shine to, 174

care tool kit, 149
damaged, 144
nutrition's role, 138
thinning, 139, 151, 181
hairbrushes, 146, 147, 149, 174
hair color, 148
haircuts, 136, 144, 146, 147
hair dryer, 146, 149, 174
hair extensions, 140–42
Hair2wear, 140–41, 196
Hanky Panky thongs, 166, 197
heavy cream, substitutes, 59
High-Heel Workout, 76
Hopson, Maury, 146, 196
hormone replacement therapy, 182
humidifiers, 88
hyaluronic acid, 112, 132

Inglot Cosmetics Freedom System
palettes, 125, 196
ingredient substitutes, 58–59
injuries, 66–67, 68
inner peace, 20

jeans, 159, 160, 162, 165, 173
Jergens BB Body Perfecting Skin Cream,
90, 194

kale, 30, 33, 37, 39, 41
kale chips, 33
Kérastase Resistance Ciment Thermique,
174, 197
KeVita Sparkling Probiotic Drink, 175, 197
Kevyn Aucoin products, 109, 110, 111, 113,
115, 195

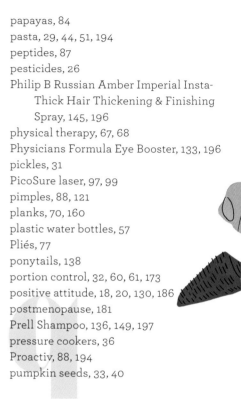
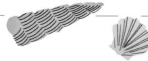

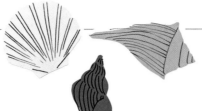

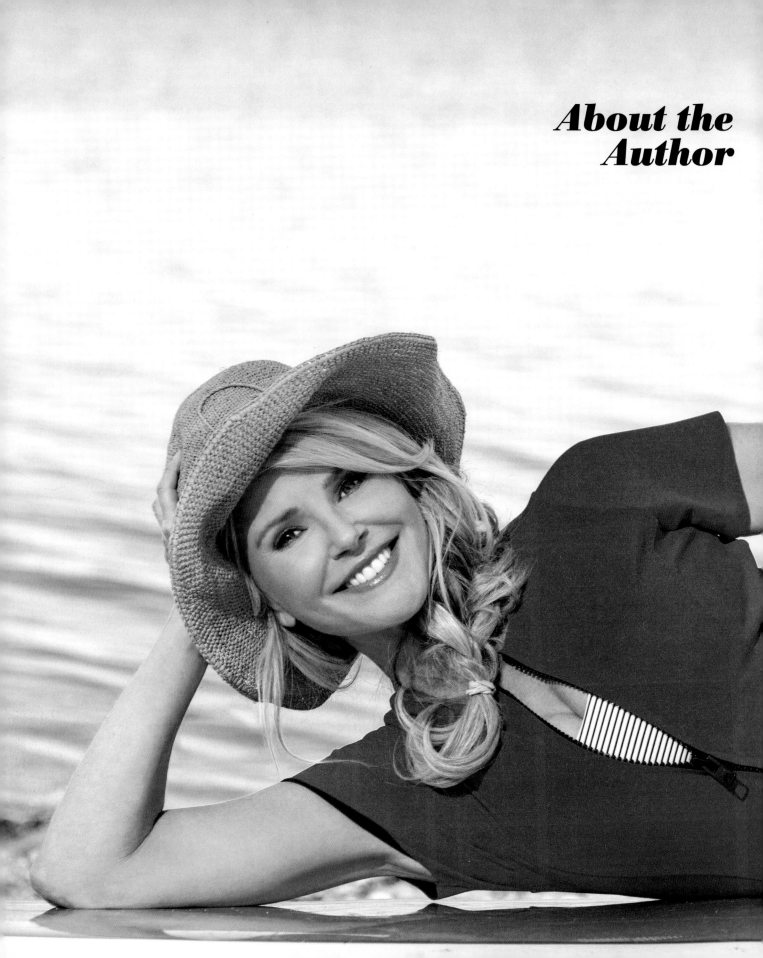

About the Author

Christie Brinkley has appeared on more than five hundred magazine covers and gained worldwide fame in the seventies with three consecutive years of *Sports Illustrated* swimsuit issue covers. She spent twenty-five years as the face of CoverGirl in the longest-running cosmetics contract held by any model in history, and has also contracted with other major brands. Brinkley has gone from "Breck Girl" to "Uptown Girl" to the girl in the red Ferrari in the classic *Vacation* films, and is now a household brand name with her Christie Brinkley Authentic Skincare, her Hair2wear Christie Brinkley Collection of fashionable hair extensions and wigs, and her Christie Brinkley Eyewear. She partnered with Total Gym, which has been one of the bestselling producers of total-body fitness equipment in the United States for the past twenty years.

Brinkley has been featured several times in *People* magazine's "World's Most Beautiful" issues, and was most recently on the cover of the magazine when she celebrated her sixtieth birthday. She starred on Broadway and London's West End in productions of *Chicago,* and had cameos on several TV shows, including a recurring role on NBC's *Parks and Recreation.* She is also an artist, writer, photographer, designer, philanthropist, and environmentalist. Brinkley lives in Sag Harbor, New York, and is the proud mother of three amazing artists in their own right.

*Spread sunshine and joy,
life's too short for anything else*

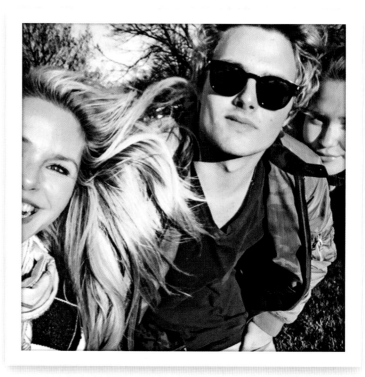

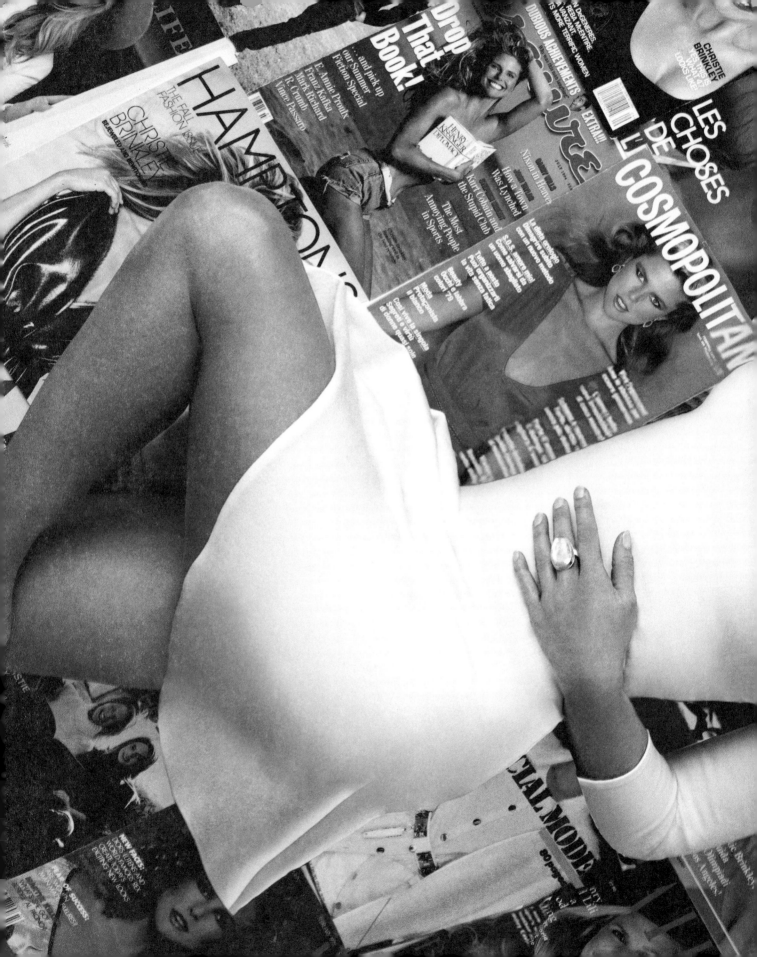